Way of the Heart

Walter Lübeck

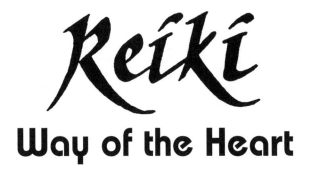

Way of the Heart

The Reiki Path of Initiation
A Wonderful Method for Inner Development and
Holistic Healing

LOTUS LIGHT
SHANGRI-LA

Disclaimer

Reiki is an effective system for healing and stimulating mental, emotional, and spiritual growth. However, Reiki does not make the visit to a doctor, naturopath, or psychotherapist superfluous when there is a suspicion of a serious health disorder. Naturopathy (which also includes Reiki) would like to supplement orthodox medicine wherever the latter cannot heal people and animals, but it does not want to consider it unnecessary in any respect.

The information and exercises introduced in my book have been carefully researched and passed on to the best of my knowledge and conscience. Despite this fact, the author and the publisher do not assume any type of liability for damages of any type which occur through the direct or indirect application or utilization of the statements in this book.

A further note: The illustrations in this book show nude people in order to graphically demonstrate the hand positions of Reiki and better convey the atmosphere of closeness, freedom, and love which Reiki radiates. But this does not mean that Reiki must be practiced in the nude. Participants in the Reiki training seminars are also fully dressed.

When I talk about the Master, Grand Master, and students, the feminine form of these words is fundamentally included as well. When the word "he" is used in place of the more awkward "he or she," it is not meant to be discriminatory in any way.

1st English edition 1996
© by Lotus Light Publications
Box 325, Twin Lakes, WI 53181
The Shangri-La Series is published in cooperation
with Schneelöwe Verlagsberatung, Federal Republic of Germany
© 1990 reserved by Windpferd Verlagsgesellschaft mbH, Aitrang
All rights reserved
Translated by Christine M. Grimm
Coverillustration by Roland Tietsch
Cover design by Wolfgang Jünemann
Overall production: Schneelöwe, D-87648 Aitrang
ISBN 0-941524-91-4

Printed in the USA

Dedication

For Manuela

Table of Contents

Preface

In the beginning God created the heavens and the earth. The earth was without form and void, and darkness was upon the face of the deep; and the spirit of God was moving over the face of the waters. And God said: "Let there be light"; and there was light.

This is how the first three verses of the story of Creation read. Many people have already tried to interpret Genesis, yet it has always just remained an attempt because any one person can only formulate an interpretation in so far as his level of perception permits. The true depths of this story will probably remain a secret for a very long time to come. Or will they?

How is the story of Creation related to this book in front of you? In his texts, the author also uses such terms as God, light, life energy, energy transference to matter, and successfully attempts to explain the Reiki energy. The fronts of ideology are built on these few concepts. This is the point where things end for the old scientific way of thinking and where the search starts for the new spirit of the times. For most people, such things are currently as inexplicable as the story of Creation.

In the author's opinion, the fundamental quality of Reiki is truth and divine—which means all-embracing—love and perception. All people aspire to pure truth and love within the depths of their hearts, making this book a wonderful challenge for a person to take this one path from among the multitude of paths. The author answers many questions that are posed time and again in daily practice as well. I find the open communication of information, even about uncomfortable questions like Reiki and money, one's own aggressions, claims to power, and why I want to have a Reiki initiation, to be quite positive.

The path of Reiki is one possibility of directly feeling the love of God. Intellectual explanations regarding energy or love are no longer necessary because they simply exist. Yet, all people must experience this on their own. Together with my wife, I received the first Reiki initiation five years ago and we have had many deep personal experiences since then. I could now list a wealth of examples describing the experiences of many members of the "Reiki Help-Ring," but they must be experienced personally in order to overcome doubt. However, it is only possible

11

for me to have personal experiences when I live, and living means being in motion. Otherwise, my life will be lived for me and I cannot control what moves me. The masses of humanity have already let themselves be moved for much too long, and this is why each of us bears a share of the burden for the destruction of the planet Earth with us. If we could only finally comprehend that each bit of matter is more than just simply matter and the whole is more than the sum of the individual components, it would be much easier for us to understand energies like that of Reiki.

May this book give you an impulse to be ready for new experiences in order to gradually free yourself from this state of having your life lived for you.

Hans-Jürgen Regge
Founder of the Reiki Help-Association

Hamburg, December 30, 1990

Acknowledgements

I thank the many people who see the world in a different way than I do and did and still the courage to discuss their points of view with me. As a result, you have helped me to see and experience the many facets of the Creation.

With relation to this book, I am particularly obliged to thank Renate Lorke and Wolfgang Grabowski, who helped me get my feet on the ground and my consciousness in my heart during my growth processes. I would like to thank Manfred Steiner, my Chinese-boxing master, for showing me that spirituality without practical use is worthless and for exemplifying how a Master teaches by how he lives own life. My gratitude as well to: Phyllis Lei Furumoto for her example of loving, unifying strength; Brigitte Müller, my Reiki Master, for the many impulses for thought and feeling; Vera Suchanek, who showed me how it is when a person radiates love; and my cat companions in life, Cinderella and Bagheera, for their liveliness and willfulness.

Introduction to the Revised and Expanded 6th Edition

Much has happened since the year 1990 in which I wrote the manuscript for *Reiki—The Path of the Heart*. The *Usui System of Natural Healing* has spread at a tremendous speed and will soon be just as familiar to the general public as autogenous training or yoga. Since then, there have been a series of new developments, and many different views on Reiki and the Reiki tradition have arisen. This is hardly a surprise since there are more than 10,000 Reiki teachers throughout the world living at least that many different facets of the Reiki path. These events have moved me to revise this current book and expand it with information on important relevant points. Among other things, there is now information on various Reiki organizations and explanations of new developments. One section has also been dedicated to my checklist for the minimum standards of Reiki training in all three traditional degrees, as well as the ethical guidelines for the work of a Reiki Master-teacher. In recent years, this information has proved to be a very useful help in decision-making for Reiki students of all degrees. It is hardly possible for the non-initiated to realistically evaluate the diversity of seminars offered without this type of support.

It is important for me to comment that all of the views published in this book have evolved from almost seven yours of practice as a Reiki teacher, my intensive research, and many thousands of Reiki sessions and personal consultations, but they are naturally not meant to represent "ultimate truths," and cannot fulfill this function. The contents of this book have proved to be very useful in the practice. Yet, like anything which human beings have thought up and put to practice, it can naturally still be improved, supplemented, and perhaps at some time even replaced by something completely different that functions even better. In this sense, please use my opinions as contributions to the discussion and stimulation for thought. And don't be too angry with me if my perspective deviates too much from your own in one point or another. When discussed by people with an open mind, different opinions can accelerate development. On the other hand, cultivating one-sidedness means standstill and the obstruction of evolution. In my experience, flexibility, love, and tolerance in particular are very important qualities when we deal with Reiki. Rules and traditions should exist for the sake of people and not the other way around. Still, it is very important to thoroughly examine the circumstances before declaring time-tested structures and traditional knowledge to be superfluous and consigning it to the scrap-heap.

I would be very pleased to receive feedback on this book. But please understand that I will not necessarily be able to respond in writing. More than one hundred letters from all parts of the world turn up at my home every week and it's hard for me to even keep up with reading them—to say nothing of answering them. This is also a development I could have hardly imagined in the year 1990...

And now I would like to wish you much enjoyment with the new, expanded *Reiki—The Path of the Heart*.

Walter Lübeck

Introduction

During the years in which I intensively became involved with and examined the Usui System of Reiki, it became increasingly clear to me that Reiki can be a wonderful path for self-discovery and development of the personality.

In the holistic, natural sense, Reiki energy stimulates the body to heal. It helps free blocked emotional energies, such as those which have been built up in the form of an armor of muscle, once again making them available to the individual. Reiki helps by triggering an intensive process of purification that, when it is supported by healthy nutrition, can initiate deep-reaching organic processes of rejuvenation. These two effects are the preconditions for the following "filling" of the bodily structure with the universal life energy, helping trigger growth processes on all levels.

In my Reiki Handbook, these two processes stood in the foreground. Before comprehensive spiritual development can take place, the body must become healthy, making it strong enough for these challenges. On the other hand, the body cannot be healed on a lasting basis if the spirit is not fundamentally healed. The concept of the "spirit" has a different meaning in Asian medicine and philosophy than in the Western world. This term is understood as the deep longing for self-realization, the desire for relationships with other people, meaningful work, tenderness, joy, and procreation (in both the literal and figurative sense). In essence, this is the longing for unconditional participation in the vital processes which the creative force has provided for us on the material level of existence. Qualities like thankfulness, love, consciousness, responsibility for oneself, respect, and hope, as well as the survival instinct, belong to a healthy spirit. This book then is concerned with the healing of the spirit and at the same time, because it is closely associated with it, the fundamentals of spiritual development with Reiki.

The sequence of the procedure on the Reiki path is very similar to that of traditional yoga training. In this old spiritual tradition as well, the healing of the physical level, for example, through Asanas (body work), Pranayama (breathing work), and didactic conversations about healthful thought and proper lifestyle, are introduced in order to slowly lead up to spiritual development. Although the Reiki path has many aspects which clearly differentiate it from yoga, the underlying structures are the same. Both attempt to bring the human being into contact with God.

Beyond practical involvement with the universal life energy, those who not only want to become familiar with the healthful effects of Reiki power on the physical level but also feel themselves attracted to Reiki, the path of healing love as a method of personality development, will also need to become inwardly involved with the principles of love, freedom, responsibility for oneself, truth, and the laws of growth-promoting energy exchange (see 3rd chapter).

Mikao Usui perceived the importance of these mental and spiritual teachings and processes of becoming healthy quite quickly after the first practical experiences with the healing Reiki power. He then established the five life principles that have been passed on to this day, as well as the three rules of healing (see Chapters One and Three).

At the beginning, I had difficulty with understanding and applying the meaning and use of these short sentences. Only later did I gradually discover the deep wisdom of the principles for spiritual orientation on the Reiki path. My experience with the fundamental possibilities of mental and spiritual development for the three Reiki degrees was similar. Each of them offers you a very special stimulation for growth and addresses its own themes. If you involve yourself with them, gather experiences, and accept your own standpoint and yourself with time, you will create a foundation of learning possibilities for the next degree. You can naturally also do the Second Degree without having taken full advantage of the first as an opportunity for the development of your personality. The initiation always works.

However, rushing from initiation to initiation without any longer pauses to develop the personality with the newly acquired means tends to result in a step backwards. The problems of life cannot be mastered through initiations. These can only create the preconditions for taking part in an extensive training and then returning to the game of life with better cards, taking the path, and attending to the necessary work with improved tools.

Reiki can also be used as a holistic, natural method of healing and relaxation without the need for you to open up to conscious processes of self-discovery. The Reiki techniques and energies are also effective in this manner. However, in this case Reiki is "just" a very effective method of healing for the physical body. The more extensive processes of development can only be revealed to you if you become involved with your mental and spiritual structures, which are naturally different in every person. Reiki supports this individuality and helps you find your very own path. But you must walk the path yourself.

Reiki, yoga, methods of meditation, and other techniques help each person to live, but they do not replace life itself. A person who has no experiences cannot work through them. Someone who is not curious about the world will be incapable of learning anything. Those who hang on to old patterns will not grow. There are no magic formulas like "Illumination in 30 Days with Reiki." But there is already a red thread which goes through all the degrees and to which the students of the various initiation levels can orient themselves.

It is my intention to show you what I know of the Reiki path and what I have learned from it in order to stimulate you in your own development. I think it is easier to take a path for which you have received a sketch than one you know nothing about.

If you are considering opening yourself up to this path, take your time in reading this book and give some thought to my viewpoints. Think about what could happen for you and try it out. In no case should you attempt to just orient yourself on my opinions. Then you would just have many empty doctrines about Reiki in your head. Involve yourself with the thoughts on the individual degrees and don't forget to put it all back together again when you're done.

In case you already have a Reiki Degree, compare your experiences and the conclusions that you have drawn with mine. Perhaps (I hope) there is something important for you here. The exercises will possibly help you to better understand an aspect of your personality, learn to love it, and therefore become a bit more free.

The three most important energies in the Reiki system are those of truth, love, and freedom. Everything that can lead you to these can in some way be compatible with the Reiki force. Yet, for me the most important essence of these three energies is love, the love of God who has given us the freedom to have our own experiences and thereby contribute to the living growth of the universe in its entirety.

I have acquired my ideas about the Reiki path through my experiences with the three degrees, various forms of meditation, inner martial arts like Tai Chi Ch'uan and Aikido, and certain spiritual experiences which have very much influenced me. The long years of group and individual therapy have helped me see my experiences with somewhat less transfigured eyes and perceiving the power games that I play when talking about them. Of the many paths with which I have been permitted to become familiar, Reiki has proved to be the most suitable one for me. I wouldn't want to be without it and hope that it will give you experiences that are similar to mine in their beauty. This is one of the most important reasons for the creation of this book. Another reason is helping myself on the path by writing down what I have experienced with Reiki.

If you like, this book is a type of journal of my own development. Now I want to wish you much enjoyment in reading and feeling your way into the Reiki path of healing love.

Your

Walter Lübeck

Chapter One

What is Reiki?

Before I go into more detail about Reiki as a path of self-realization, I would like to relate something about the past of the Reiki movement, as well as some results of scientific research on this energy and describe a few important experiences with Reiki. As I see it, the special qualities of the Reiki path can be better understood with this approach.

"Historical" Reiki has existed for many thousands of years. Buddha and probably Jesus healed with it as well. In Tibet and India there are suggestions of Reiki in the history of spiritual knowledge. There are various forms of healing by the laying on of hands under names like "Buddha Hand" and "medical Buddha practice" in this cultural region. It is interesting to note that initiation is imparted through an authorized teacher, at least on the higher levels of competence for these methods. Mantras and symbols also played an important role in this process as "tools."

Some of the areas of the Second Degree and the Master knowledge suggest the conclusion that the Kahunas of Polynesia worked with Reiki. From there, but also from India, the traces can be followed back to Egypt and Central Asia, among other places. Various signs indicate that the origin of the traditions from which Dr. Mikao Usui, the first modern Reiki Grand Master, developed his Usui System of "Natural Healing" may have ultimately been formed in the highly developed culture of Lemuria (Mu), a continent which sunk in the Pacific after a world-wide catastrophe many ages ago.

The transference of practical spiritual abilities through initiations, given by people who are trained for this purpose, also exists in other spiritual systems today. Examples of this are Kriya yoga, transcendental meditation, the transference of Shakipad for the awakening of the kundalini for the yogis, and also the Sufis, whose initiation is called the "transference of Baraka." In Christianity, baptism and communion are examples of initiations.

The personal developments resulting from this vary greatly, as do the powers which are transferred. The common denominator seems to be that, from the very foundations of his being, a person can get closer to God. This act of getting closer cannot be achieved through exercises or privations. It is God's help which is given to us and which we human beings need in order to come into direct contact with God when we have decided to seek the divine presence.

These initiations are then basically a gift. In the New Testament, the meaning of initiations becomes clear in the baptism of Jesus by John the Baptist. Jesus did not actually need this transference of energy. He was the Son of God. Yet, he still requested the blessing of baptism of his own free will. Only through this decision was Jesus blessed with the Holy Spirit, because he independently decided to seek a close relationship to God.

This decision is important and comprehendible for every human being. We are all children of God, but our will is free. If you make the decision to be close to God with your independent will, you initiate a deep-reaching transformation of your self as a result. You create a conscious unity with the universe and the source of love and light. Afterwards, life is usually as it was before, yet you feel the close relationship to God in your heart. This will cause a permanent change in the way you see the world and live in it. A further piece of heaven comes down to earth through this decision.

This short excursion into history which has long passed, and to similar systems, will perhaps give you some impulses for your own inquires and reflections.

The story of Reiki deals with the rediscovery of the practical use of the Reiki energy in our age. It tells of completely normal people, their questions and worries. None of the Reiki Grand Masters were healers or illuminated people. But each of them helped to give love and light more opportunities to develop in our age. Each of them gave what they could and passed on the knowledge with their efforts. I am thankful to them because many people, including myself, would not have had such an easy and certain access to the universal life energy today without them.

The History of the Usui System of Reiki

At the end of the nineteenth century, the Reiki system was rediscovered by the Christian priest Dr. Mikao Usui in Japan. This remarkable person was born around the year 1860, attended a Christian mission school, and later studied at a preacher's seminar. Eventually he became the director of a small Christian school near Kyoto. Here young men who wanted to become preachers were trained. In addition, Usui also taught and preached there on certain occasions. One Sunday after the church service, one of his students asked him whether he believed everything that was written in the Bible. For example, did he believe that Jesus healed people simply through the laying on of hands? Usui answered that he did. The student then asked if he had personally experienced something like this, and Dr. Usui had to say he hadn't.

In response to this, Dr. Usui was told that such blind faith was probably acceptable for him as an older person. However, the student did not want to build his life and work on something which no one could prove to him. This wasn't enough for him as a young person with so many questions about life. This discussion moved Dr. Usui so much that he resigned from his office the next day and went off to seek the truth. Now he wanted to personally know where he stood and not base the rest of his life on blind faith either. His search first led him to the USA. He studied ancient languages, philosophy, the science of religion, and theory of the Bible in Chicago in order to have direct sources of information on Jesus' acts of healing revealed to him. He then also chose the topic "acts of healing in the New Testament" for his doctoral dissertation. However, despite his intensive studies, the priest received no deeper information about Jesus' methods of healing. Yet, he did find references which said Buddha also performed similar miracles.

Dr. Usui followed this trail, returned to his homeland, and visited many Buddhist monasteries in Japan in order to find clues that could lead him further in his search. Yet, every monk he asked about Buddha's abilities in terms of healing physical disorders answered that there was no longer any knowledge about this. In addition, the contemporary students of Buddha had concentrated completely on the healing of the spirit* since this was the most important thing. Without a healthy spirit, a person could never become and remain healthy. The healing of the physical body—which they felt to be secondary—was left to the physicians. At this point in time, Dr. Usui did not know how to understand this important statement. Many years later, he remembered it and understood its deeper meaning.

After years of searching, he found a Zen monastery near Kyoto that possessed the most extensive collection of old Buddhist sutras in Japan. Its abbot invited the priest to research in the library to his heart's desire. Dr. Usui did not wait to be asked twice and thankfully accepted the offer. At first, he looked at the texts written in Japanese, but couldn't find any more precise details in them. However, there were some references to older writings kept in the Chinese language which appeared to contain more information on the topic of his interest. So Dr. Usui learned the Old Chinese language and writing. However, there were only imprecise statements in the Chinese material as well. Not until the priest acquired more extensive knowledge of the Old Indic language of Sanskrit, also used by Buddha and his contemporaries, did he discover what he had been looking for. In the ancient sutras written by an unknown disciple of Gautama Buddha there was an exact description of the methods, symbols, and formulas the holy man used to heal people and how he had passed on these abilities to others.

After searching for so many years, Dr. Usui found what he had been looking for. But he was still missing one thing! Academic knowledge was not enough for him. He wanted to personally experience the healing through the laying on of hands. However, the writings were inadequate for this purpose. Although they imparted the knowledge, this did not include the power to turn it into reality. He spoke with the abbot of the monastery, who had become his friend in the meantime, about this last difficulty. The monk advised him to go to the holy mountain of Kurayama, which was 25 kilometers away, in order to meditate and fast in a special manner. He should trust in God to give him access to the healing power.

At the same time, the monk warned Dr. Usui because he feared

---

*Compare with my comments on this in the introduction.

the priest might lose his life in the attempt. Mikao Usui decided to risk this last step as well and went to the place of power in order to fast, meditate, and pray. This meditation lasted 21 days, and what he had prayed for actually occurred on the last day: a bright ray of light came down to him from heaven, struck his forehead, and filled him with strength and vitality. All the weakness and stiffness produced by the long period of meditation fell away from him. In a quick succession, he saw symbols that he had already encountered in the old Sanskrit text shrouded in shining energy bubbles. They imprinted themselves in his mind for all time and activated his access to the universal life energy.

After this experience, the old priest stood up and began the long descent. Along the way, he injured his foot on a rock, providing the first opportunity of trying out the new powers. And they actually worked: after he had held his hands over the injury for some minutes, the bleeding and pain subsided so that he could continue on his way.

When Dr. Usui arrived at the foot of the mountain, he went into a little inn and ordered a large meal for himself. As the innkeeper's daughter brought his meal, he noticed that the girl was crying. Her cheek was swollen, and she had a terrible toothache. Dr. Usui asked whether he would be permitted to help her, putting his hands on the afflicted spot after she had consented. Some time later, the young woman's pain had eased and the swelling subsided. After finishing his meal with great relish, Dr. Usui returned to the monastery in order to tell his friend, the abbot, about his experiences and discuss further proceedings. When the priest arrived, he found the old man bedridden with a bad case of arthritis. Once again, the priest was able to help with Reiki and soothe the pains of the afflicted person. During the following days, the two deliberated about what would be the best thing to do with this new, wonderful ability. They ultimately came to the conclusion that it would be best to use Reiki to help people who were no longer capable of taking care of themselves because of illness and had to live in poverty for this reason.

Afterwards, Dr. Usui spent many years with the beggars in the slums of Kyoto. He healed many of them through the Reiki energy and then sent them back into life so that they could work and take care of themselves and their relatives. However, some time later, he saw the people who he had healed sitting back on

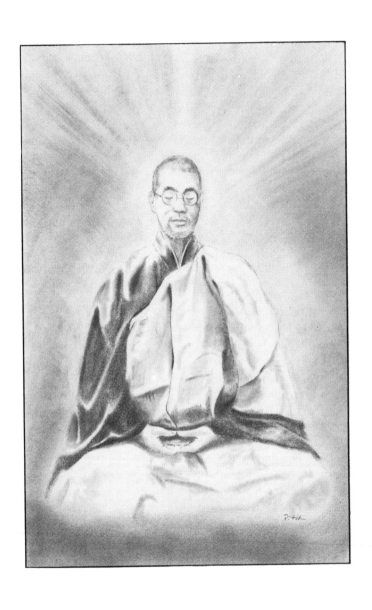

*After 21 days of meditating and fasting, Dr. Mikao Usui
received the gift of becoming a Reiki channel.*

the street and begging again. In response to his question about how life was for them now, they gave a similar response time and again: they were doing well, they were healthy, but it was so unpleasant and strenuous to take care of themselves and work. They felt better when they begged. They did not have to bear responsibility and it was nice to live from other people's prosperity. These reactions to his efforts saddened Dr. Usui very much. He realized that it is not enough to physically heal a person. The spirit must also be included in the healing process. Under the impression of his experiences in the slums of Kyoto, he formulated three principles for holistic healing:

1. First heal the spirit*
2. Then heal the body.
3. Beggars** know no gratitude.

During this period of his life, Dr. Usui probably came to understand the correlations between illness and learning processes, the value of health, the purpose of one's own responsibility, gratitude, and the laws of energy exchange. He wrote down what he had learned in order to share his perceptions with later generations as well and made sure that every student receives instruction in this matter when he receives the First Degree initiation. The five Reiki principles of life are therefore still an important part of the initiation seminars today, and every student receives a copy of them in order to grapple with their content. The life principles are:

1. Don't get angry—just for today.
2. Don't worry—just for today.
3. Earn your daily bread honestly.
4. Try to be kind to all living beings around you.
5. Be thankful for the many blessings.

---

* Please see my comments on the meaning of the term "spirit" in the Introduction.
**Within this context, "beggars" are people whose mental attitude is geared towards taking from others without giving them any type of appropriate service in return.

The thought that no one can truly become healthy if his health is not of value to him and that everyone should provide a return service for the initiations into the Reiki Degrees and for Reiki treatments has been passed down from Reiki Master to Reiki Master since Dr. Usui's time. Even today, it still forms an important component of the traditional Reiki training. Afterwards, Mikao Usui spent many years in Japan teaching and training students in the methods of transferring Reiki.

Unfortunately, we do not know much about his life. Most of what we do know is based on oral traditions. Perhaps we will learn more when there is once again a connection to the Reiki movement in Japan or Korea (see below). Dr. Usui died at the end of the 1920s. Up to that time, he had trained 18 Master students* and received a high distinction for his work from Tenno, the Japanese Emperor. His ashes found their resting place in a Zen temple in Tokyo.

Dr. Usui's two children did not want to work with Reiki on a full-time basis, and the Grand Master office of the Usui Shiki Ryoho (Usui System of Natural Healing) was therefore passed on to the physician and retired Marine commander Dr. Chujiro Hayashi.

Hayashi came from a family of the Japanese upper class and was Usui's student for many years. In 1925, he was initiated into the Degree of Reiki Master at the age of 47 years by the rediscoverer of the Reiki method. The doctor set up a clinic in Tokyo, close to the Emperor's palace, which he called Shina No Machi. Treatment was provided here for all types of minor and severe diseases with Reiki and special diets. Every day, the 16 Reiki Practitioners whom he had trained were there to give healing sessions at the eight couches in a large therapy room. Most of the patients at this clinic came from the class of the aristocracy and high society. Dr. Hayashi systematized the Reiki training, researched optimal forms of treatment, and prepared many reports on the effects of Reiki based on his experiences.

Among other things, he drew up a plan for the whole-body treatment and discovered that Reiki always automatically flows

---

*It is often said that Dr. Usui did not differentiate between the three degrees, but this part of the oral tradition probably permits the conclusion that the founder of the Reiki method imparted at least the Master Degree separately.

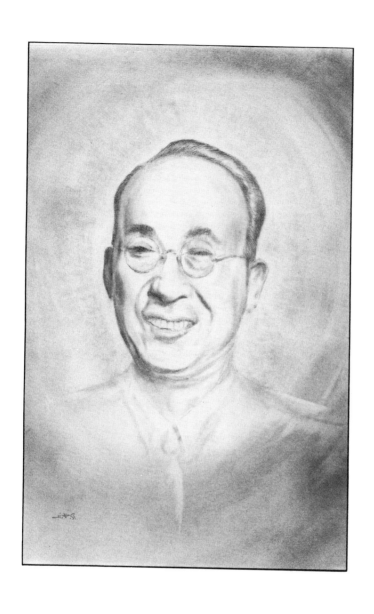

The second Grand Master of Reiki, Dr. Chujiro Hayashi

to where it is needed. There are some misunderstandings about this statement, which I would like to clear up here. It is absolutely important where the hands of the person giving the treatment are laid during a Reiki session. Otherwise, Dr. Hayashi would hardly have developed his form of systematic whole-body treatment practiced and taught in his clinic. Although Reiki is drawn in by the body, it must first break down many blocks in a process which is often quite protracted until the energy can flow directly and within the short amount of time from the sole of the foot to the liver, for example. From my research I know that the large joints—hips, knees, ankles—must frequently first be provided with adequate Reiki before the universal life energy can find its way from the lower end of the body to the upper end.

Dr. Hayashi's statement can be understood to mean that Reiki is always attracted to zones with disharmonious structure and develops its effect there. In accordance with this, perfectly healthy tissue does not attract Reiki. In addition, probably every person who gives treatment with Reiki (over a longer period of time) becomes familiar with the effect that Reiki hands have the urge to "want" to go to the afflicted regions of the body and practically stay "glued" to it. In this case, the person giving the treatment feels something like a strong aversion to removing his hands from this spot. This is why the Reiki training also teaches its students: "When in doubt, trust your hands!"

Unfortunately, we no longer have access to Dr. Hayashi's writings today. Shortly before Japan entered into World War II, Dr. Hayashi passed on the office of Grand Master to Hawayo Takata, a Japanese woman who lived on Hawaii and had been healed from severe cancer at his hospital, where she found her way to Reiki. Mrs. Takata had lost her husband when she was 29 years old and had to take care of her two small children alone. This is never an easy task for anyone and was particularly difficult to do at this time.

When Hawayo Takata was 35 years old, she had all possible diseases: appendicitis, a benign tumor, gallstones, and, as the last straw, she had asthma and could not be operated on under a general anesthetic. She had also lost weight and finally went down to just 97 pounds. Many of her relatives had died during the past year, so that she had less and less help with her problems and suffered from depression. During this difficult time, it was only her love for her children that kept her from committing suicide. Mrs. Takata also went to church on a regular basis and meditated in order to receive help from God.

One day, when she absolutely no longer had any idea of how to cope with her life, she cried out to God after meditating. She prayed that she no longer knew what to do and asked for help for herself and her small children. She thought that God would certainly help her after hearing her prayer. Suddenly, she heard a voice telling her three times that she should first cure her physical diseases. Then all other problems would also be solved.

Three weeks later, one of her sisters died. Mrs. Takata took on the difficult task of bringing the sad news to her parents, who were on a longer visit in Japan to the ancestral home of the family in Yamaguchi. Both daughters accompanied Mrs. Takata on the this trip. On this occasion, she also wanted to bring the ashes of her husband to the Ohtani temple in Japan in order to pay him final honors and then visit a hospital in Tokyo, the Maeda Orthopedic Clinic which belonged to a friend of the family, so that she could undergo treatment. When the doctor saw her, he shook his head and said that she first would have to regain her strength before considering the possibility of an operation. So Mrs. Takata and her daughters remained in the hospital. Some weeks later, Dr. Maeda found her to be in good enough condition for an operation and had preparations made.

However, while she was being prepared for the operation, she again heard the voice that had already spoken to her on Hawaii. This time it told her that the operation was unnecessary! Incredulously, she pinched herself in the arm. But she wasn't dreaming. Only after the voice had imparted the message three times did she believe it. She stood up and told the confused nurses that she now did not want to an operation. The women were understandably quite alarmed and quickly got Dr. Maeda so that he could clarify the situation. Mrs. Takata explained to the concerned physician that she was not afraid of dying during the operation, but would very much like to know if there wasn't some other possibility for her to become healthy. Dr. Maeda thought about this for a while and then asked whether she wanted to remain in Japan for long. When he heard that she planned a visit of two years, he sent her to his sister, Mrs. Shimura, who was a dietician in his hospital.

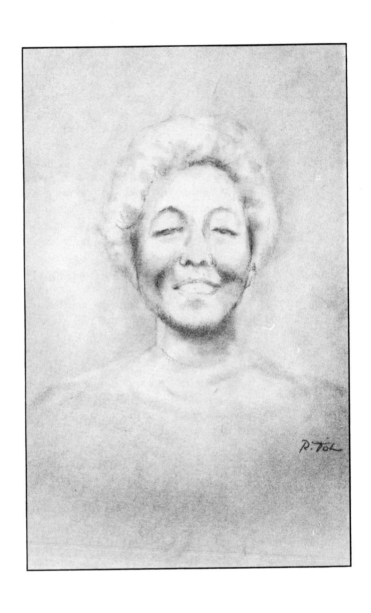

Mrs. Hawayo Takata, the third Grand Master of Reiki

In the following conversation with her, Mrs. Takata heard of the wondrous healing through the Reiki Master Chujiro Hayashi, who had revived Mrs. Shimura from a deep coma after all the medical skills had been applied in vain. Soon afterwards, Hawayo Takata was brought to Dr. Hayashi's clinic. The Reiki Master attended to her and had her treated with the universal life energy by two initiated colleagues for many hours a day during the following six months.

She returned to the Maeda Hospital on a regular basis to have her recuperation confirmed by orthodox medical means and permit any possible complications to be recognized in due time. In addition to the transferences of Reiki, she was given a special diet which essentially consisted of sunflower seeds, red-beet juice, grapefruit, almonds, and other fresh fruits and vegetables.

She found the sessions to be quite strange. Dr. Hayashi's assistants silently laid their hands on her body, and after a short time she felt a pleasant, strong warmth on the places treated. Curious, she examined her bed and the floor when no one was in the room, but was unable to find any concealed machines that could have caused these strange sensations. One day, during a session she could no longer restrain herself and reached into the wide sleeve of the Practitioner's traditional kimono. The man was surprised, but thought she needed handkerchiefs and gave her some. Mrs. Takata refused them and, in an agitated state, asked where the batteries and the heating device were. Both practitioners looked at each other in astonishment and then broke into loud laughter.

His attention attracted by the noise, Dr. Hayashi looked into the room. In response to her questions, he told the amazed woman about Reiki, the universal life energy directed into her afflicted body by the laying on of hands. After this important event, Hawayo Takata's interest in this wonderful power was awakened. She talked with Dr. Hayashi about it time and again, informing him of her desire to become his student. This was an unusual privilege for someone who had not grown up in Japan; and despite her efforts, she would have hardly been accepted into a Reiki course had not the famous internist Dr. Maeda, who also was Hayashi's uncle, written a letter of recommendation for Takata.

Later, after her health had been completely restored, she was initiated into the First Degree of the Usui System of Natural Healing in a four-day seminar and carefully trained in the fundamentals of its competent application. Dr. Hayashi's program of instruction was designed as follows: The first day was dedicated to treatment of the head and the throat, understanding of the disorders that frequently occur there, and the method of treating them with Reiki. On the second day, the treatment of the chest, stomach, and abdomen was demonstrated to her and the occurring diseases of this region discussed. The main topic on the third day was the back, and the doctor explained the use of Reiki in acute health problems and accidents of all types on the fourth day. During this last portion of the seminar, Dr. Hayashi also commented in detail on the spiritual aspect of the Usui System of Natural Healing, referring to the principles of life and healing established by Dr. Usui. The Grand Master put special emphasis on the principle that every illness, whether it is of a physical or emotional and mental nature, has a cause and that a Reiki Practitioner must heal this cause of disharmony through treatment with the universal life energy. Only then will all of the symptoms based on this cause also disappear. As an aid in their practical work with Reiki, Dr. Hayashi gave his students a list of health disorders and their possible causes.*

Hawayo Takata stayed for more than one year with the Reiki doctor and continued to be trained by him. Dr. Hayashi required practical training of about one year's length in his clinic from all his students, which most of them fulfilled as a secondary occupation. The Hawaiian woman's earnestness and deep interest in Reiki and healing moved the Grand Master to initiate her into the Second Degree, the Practitioner Degree.

Mrs. Takata later returned to Hawaii with the gift of healing and treated many people there with the Reiki energy.

Some weeks later, Takata received a visit. Chujiro Hayashi and his daughter had come to give her further training. During

*It is frequently said that no written information about Reiki should be disseminated. On the basis of my practice of Reiki and the facts I have learned about the history of Reiki, I cannot agree with this opinion. Dr. Usui studied old Sanskrit writings, without which there would have been no Usui System of Natural Healing spread throughout the world today, and Dr. Hayashi gave his students of the First Degree written accompanying information.

the course of several months, the doctor conveyed to her further knowledge about Reiki, held courses, and then initiated her to be a Reiki Master on February 22, 1938. Soon afterwards, the father and daughter returned to Japan.

Hawayo Takata did much in the following years to spread Reiki on Hawaii. She established a Reiki center in which she lived with her family, treated the ill, and introduced receptive people to the Usui System of Reiki. In addition, she travelled much on the islands and held Reiki courses since increasingly more people had heard of the woman with healing hands and wanted to learn her method. At the beginning of the year 1940, as Japan increasingly approached the point of war with the USA, Dr. Hayashi sensed this. He felt that after the long years in the service of healing he could no longer directly or indirectly take part in a war. On the other hand, as a Japanese from an old, traditional family, it was not possible for him to refuse active duty. So he chose a typically Japanese solution for his dilemma; he put his affairs in order and prepared himself for departure from this world.

During these days, Mrs. Takata had a dream that very much plagued her. In it, she saw that something was wrong with Dr. Hayashi and immediately travelled—as quickly as she could—to Japan to help him. After her arrival, the doctor confirmed her concerns and both of them spent many days in serious discussions about the coming war, its outcome, and the arrangements that had to be made to ensure Hawayo Takata's safety and protect the Reiki tradition. Dr. Hayashi had very clear visions of the coming events and was able to give his student much valuable advice as a result.

Soon afterwards, he called together all his friends, relatives, and the Japanese Reiki Masters, naming Mrs. Takata to be his successor for the office of Grand Master. Then, dressed in a traditional Japanese garment, he left his body forever through the strength of his will on May 10, 1941. He was laid in state for a week at the Reiki clinic Shina No Machi in Tokyo, and many Japanese from all parts of the country paid him their last respects. During this time, his body showed no symptoms of decay. Dr. Hayashi had 13 Master students.

Hawayo Takata returned to her homeland and survived the following years, particularly difficult for Americans of Japanese origin, quite well.

The guidance of her teacher helped her and made the steady continuation of the Reiki tradition possible in the West. Since this time, Mrs. Takata taught Reiki on Hawaii, in the continental USA, Canada, and South America. She trained more than 20 Masters. Before her death, she transferred the task of heading the Reiki movement to both her granddaughter Phyllis Lei Furumoto and Dr. Barbara Weber. After almost a year of working together, the paths of Mrs. Furumoto and Dr. Weber parted for personal reasons. Both founded their own organizations, the A.I.R.A. (Dr. Barbara Weber) and the Reiki Alliance (P.L. Furumoto).

At the beginning of the Eighties, Reiki then came to Europe through Brigitte Müller and has spread quickly ever since then. Even in Eastern Europe, the Usui System of Natural Healing has become quite popular. Not only since the opening of the Iron Curtain have there been local Reiki Masters here. Today (1996) there is an active exchange between Western and Eastern Reiki groups and Masters. In the disaster area around the atomic reactor in Chernobyl, Reiki Masters and Practitioners from all over the world are providing assistance, initiating people who want to do treatments, and giving Reiki to the victims of radioactive contamination. The doctors there, who have quickly learned to value Reiki because of its simple application and fantastic effects, gladly confirm the successes and promote this working relationship. In this case, the East is an example for the West.

According to information from the Reiki Masters who are active in the former republics of the Soviet Union, practitioners of orthodox medicine are much more open for subtle healing methods and also make a personal commitment to them. Reiki is not seen as competition here, but rather as a welcome supplement to orthodox medicine.

According to the newest information, there are independent lines of Reiki in both Japan and Korea. Reiki was brought to Korea by one of Dr. Hayashi's daughters, who married there. As far as I know, there are currently no direct contacts to the Korean or Japanese Reiki Masters. However, some European, American, and Australian Reiki Master initiations have already taken place in Japan and other countries of Asia. Perhaps we will eventually come into contact with the roots of the Usui System of Natural Healing in this manner. Today, there are dozens of small and medium-sized Reiki Master organizations in Europe and the USA, as well as some groups which are also open to students of the First and Second Degrees. The Reiki Alliance (Cataldo, ID) is currently the largest and fastest growing Reiki Master association with more than 1,000 members. It is internationally active and holds worldwide meetings every year alternately on the American and European continents. Hundreds of Reiki teachers come to these congresses and exchange experiences with each other, discuss relevant problems, celebrate, and enjoy the community with kindred souls sustained by Reiki.

A completely new development, which I find to be meaningful and important, is the regionalization of the Reiki Alliance. In addition to the large, international meetings, many regional and national gatherings are occurring everywhere in the world. Even Masters who are not very mobile can find and maintain contacts in this manner, become informed about new developments, or learn something from Masters who have served longer.

Somewhat parallel to the Alliance is the Reiki organization A.I.R.A., founded by the Grand Master Dr. Barbara Weber in the USA. The name later changed to T.R.T.A.I. (San Francisco, CA). In comparison to the Alliance, the opinion of the T.R.T.A.I. since about 1985 is that the Usui System of Natural Healing has seven degrees (Alliance: three degrees). Further symbols and mantras are also used. In addition, there are various differences on the general idea of the tradition, the application of the Reiki techniques, and the initiation ritual.

Other organizations mostly found in the USA and Canada, some of which are also increasingly active on the international level, are the Traditional Reiki Network (New York, NY), the Universal Masters Association (Pismo Beach, CA), The Center for Reiki Training (Southfield, MI), The Reiki Touch, Inc. (Houston, Texas), and the Reiki Plus (R) Institute (Celina, Tennessee).

In addition to Masters who are associated with the various organizations, there are also a great number of independent Reiki Masters. Which "Reiki league" a person belongs to should not be an obstacle to the contact among the groups and the members. There is already too much competitive thinking, fear of contact, and intolerance in this world. Receptive people, can always learn something at all times and everywhere.

As an aside, the organizations mentioned are purely voluntary associations of Masters who want to exchange thoughts and experiences, as well as promote mutual projects.

The terms "Grand Master" and "Reiki movement" have been mentioned quite frequently in the description of Reiki's history. In order to prevent misunderstandings, some explanations are necessary in this respect: a Reiki Grand Master essentially has the function of keeping the Reiki Masters in communication with each other, organizing meetings for the Masters, and sometimes supporting certain learning processes at the Masters' request. For these purposes, self-realization seminars are also organized for the Masters and Master students.

Moreover, the Grand Master bears the spiritual line, which means that he is responsible for the maintenance and continued existence of the respective school. The Grand Master is the spiritual center of the community of the Masters and students. In the Usui System of Natural Healing, the office of the Grand Master is transferred through the designation of the predecessor. No further initiation is necessary for this purpose. This means that no one becomes a Grand Master by way of some sort of energy transference or by way of further symbols or mantras. It is a so-called degree of competence.

Up until a few years ago, only the Grand Master initiated students into the Master Degree. In spring of 1988, Phyllis Lei Furumoto gave all Masters who felt prepared to do this official permission to also train and initiate into the Third Degree. In the Reiki movement there is fundamentally no hierarchy in which a Grand Master could exercise the function of giving instructions. Since Reiki abilities can never be lost or taken away from someone once they have been given, there are also no ways of pressuring a person to "keep him in line." A Reiki Grand Master therefore tends to be more like "the first among equals" than an authoritarian figure.

Exactly for this reason, it is not easy to be a Grand Master because the uniting power of this office is ultimately solely based on the loving power of the Grand Master's personality. If it is insufficient, then people will no longer orient themselves according to him. This means there is no Reiki guru at the top who establishes a policy line that everyone must follow, actually quite a positive practice. I think that this type of organization corresponds well to the life-promoting qualities of Reiki energy.

Membership in the individual organizations is absolutely voluntary. Those who do not wish to be members don't need to join, and there are no disadvantages for them as a result. Many Master meetings in the various organizations are even open to non-organized Masters. There are increasingly more student meetings (First and Second Degree) at which experiences and much Reiki are exchanged. There are usually also a number of Reiki Masters present as well.

The organizations of Reiki Masters usually pay for their expanses through fixed membership fees. Some organizations also offer assistance programs for Masters who are ill, have had accidents, or work in countries that are financially weak and cannot come up with the frequently high costs necessary to travel to the international Master meetings or are unable to pay the full fees. The energy of Reiki, freedom and love, can also be quickly perceived in the organizations. Just like any other situation where people unite, they naturally sometimes experience friction with each other or differences of opinion. Yet, this essentially does not obstruct the cooperation.

The same can be said for the term "Reiki movement." There is no unified Reiki movement in the sense of an organization, sect, or church. Since no Reiki student must continue the contact to his Master after a seminar or is dependent on him in any way, the possibilities for the typical mass organizations are basically quite limited.

I understand the "Reiki movement" to be all people who have been initiated into a Reiki Degree.

Scientific Information

Reiki and science? Is this really necessary? Yes, I do believe it is sometimes! In any case, it was an eye-opening experience for me when I saw two Kirlian pictures (photographic method of making visible the interplay between subtle aura energy and electro-magnetic high-tension fields) of her hands in Paula Horan's Reiki book. One of them showed them without the Reiki power and they looked completely normal, just like other people's hands. In the second picture, they were clearly brighter and surrounded by a wide, radiant halo during a distance treatment with the Second Degree.

My own search began in the rationally-oriented "corner" of our society, and this is why such directly visible proof of the Reiki power gives me something that I need. Perhaps you also need something "to hold onto" once in a while.

Beth Gray, a Reiki Master who was trained by Takata-Sensei, has discovered with the use of a very fine measuring device in cooperation with the Stanford University in California that the Reiki energy actually enters the body of the respective healer through the crown chakra. Interestingly enough, this occurs from a northerly direction in the northern hemisphere and from a southerly direction in the southern hemisphere.

Once awakened, it flows out of the hands of the Reiki channel and continues counterclockwise in the shape of a spiral. This means that its form is quite similar to that of the double helix of the DNS, the human genes. In recent years, doctors, naturopaths, and other therapists who work with Reiki have frequently received the opportunity of proving that Reiki works and that its effects are in accordance with information that has been traditionally handed down.

Perhaps there will at some time be a more extensive research project to make the many life-promoting effects of Reiki visible as well for the people who have difficulty opening up to Reiki without empirical evidence.

Using the example of scientific research on yoga and diverse methods of meditation, it can very well be seen that the result of this is spiritual disciplines meeting with much better acceptance and with fewer reservations, even from the academic community.

In view of the demands of our age, it appears to me quite desirable to also create possibilities for people without a spiritual background that make it easier for them to open up to the Reiki force and develop a personal understanding of it. The spirituality will then come on its own along with the experiences.

Experiences with the Universal Life Energy

Individuals who have already had a Reiki treatment or have even been initiated into a degree automatically encounter very personal experiences with the Reiki power. Alone the perception of the energy which occurs in both the person giving the treatment and the person receiving it during a session is so impressive that all book-learning about life-energy processes pales in comparison. To see how the flowers of a plant that just drooped sadly can stand cheerfully upright within a few hours solely through Reiki is a wonder. Things happen that appear unbelievable to someone who is not familiar with Reiki. As an example, that empty car batteries can be filled up by charging them for 20 minutes with Reiki can even be measured. However, they will quickly lose their power when the Reiki channel moves so far away from them that there is no longer contact through the aura.

Pests on house plants often fall off the infested plants over night after they have had just one Reiki treatment because the plant's powers of self-healing were supported through Reiki.

People overcome conditions of pain that have tormented them for years, can suddenly lovingly hug each other, laugh, and dance, or cure stubborn states of constipation with a few applications of Reiki.

A dog with a serious kidney disease, which the attending veterinarian had already given up on, was permanently healed within two days through Reiki. The list goes on and on, and perhaps I will do this at some point in a book on experiences with Reiki as stimulation for the development of personal applications. Yet, as impressive as these reports that have been produced as the result of contact with Reiki may be, they cannot be repeated as often as possible with precisely the same results like the experiments required by orthodox medicine.

Reiki heals completely according with holistic approaches and complies thoroughly with three individual needs of each individual while doing so. Every path of healing is then a different one, particularly for the more intensive health disorders.

In my opinion, it is particularly the emphasis on the personal needs, the exclusion of a direct influence by the Reiki channel on the path of healing and healing results that make Reiki so important and valuable. The fundamental qualities of Reiki are truth, divine—which means all-embracing—love, and perception.

Love without limitations is what we need in this transitional period in which the course of the world is still defined by the Age of Pisces, while the Age of Aquarius slowly begins to exert a new influence with a new energy. In this manner, our society can finally grow into the now absolutely necessary personal responsibility and individuality, which in time will cause the rigid power structures and mass movements of the Piscean Age to disappear. However, until that time a great deal of polluted water will flow into the oceans.

Yet, anyone who so desires can already get a foretaste of the New Age now through Reiki. Very few people will be aware of these circumstances when they become interested in Reiki since most people come to a Reiki seminar for completely different reasons, at least on the surface. The next chapter is about the path to Reiki with its questions, hopes, and fears.

Chapter Two

The Path to Reiki

Why Do People Come to Reiki?

At the beginning of every First Degree seminar I ask the participants to tell why they have come, which hopes and fears they have, and what concerns them at the moment. Time and again, they mention experiences with Reiki which move people so much that they absolutely wanted to know more and feel the power of Reiki in their own hands. There are experiences with Reiki distance healing that have initiated spontaneous healing or created changed states of consciousness similar to deep meditation. Others had been treated with Reiki because of an injury and were able to directly experience how quickly it causes wounds to heal.

The partners or close friends of people who have taken the First Degree some time ago often come as well. They are astonished as they tell of the changes that they have noticed in their friends after the initiation: that they have suddenly become more loving, open, and lively, simply making a happier impression.

Some people come because they believe the Reiki initiation will be a big step forward on their spiritual path. Others have become curious because they read a book about Reiki or heard about it from acquaintances. Many participate in a First Degree seminar because of personal difficulties in the mental and emotional or physical area. They would like to do something for their health on their own, take personal responsibility, and protect themselves from becoming seriously ill in the future.

More than 80 percent of the course participants become aware of Reiki through "word-of-mouth" propaganda. Seen statistically, this makes Reiki good tip among friends. I find this fact to be more expressive than all the explanations about the effectiveness of this energy. If it wouldn't be such a good thing, a great deal fewer people would get the idea of warmly recommending it to their friends and life partners.

I also see an increasing number of doctors, naturopaths, physiotherapists, and representatives of the medical profession and medical services in the Reiki courses. Their reasons are similar to those of the other participants, yet there is an even more important aspect more typical for the professional lives of these people: Through close contact with the many afflicted individuals, especially sensitive therapists frequently feel exhausted and virtually "drained" by their patients. This is no wonder since the ill need quite a bit of energy and frequently draw it from the open aura of the person who is treating them during contact. This naturally occurs on an unconscious level.

Even the strongest people do not survive these encounters without some type of strain. It is precisely one of the outstanding qualities of Reiki that the person initiated into it is protected from giving up his own personal energy; instead, the inexhaustible universal life energy is made available to the "energy-vampire." The afflicted person can take advantage of this to any extent desired and even does something good for the Reiki channel in the process because he also benefits from the life-promoting energy blessing. The therapist usually receives the Reiki tip from a professional colleague and then registers—with quite a bit of skepticism—for a seminar in the silent hope of this strange business being worthwhile.

Almost everyone comes with a skeptical attitude because common sense makes itself heard time and again with doubts like: "It just can't be that easy. There must be a catch somewhere!"

Fears

The fear that this is all just fraud and falsehood is probably foremost. After the experience of the first initiation this worry quickly disappears. For those who are completely skeptical and don't want to trust their own perception and the visible results, it can take longer. For me, it took almost a year before my mind also capitulated to the unending amount of evidence in favor of the existence of Reiki.

Then there is the fear of possibly becoming enslaved to a sect, church, magic society, or similar "ghastly" groups. But since there is a very cheerful and free atmosphere in the First Degree seminars and the moment in which the guru is worshipped simply never comes and no one must undress in either an emotional or physical sense, the certainty and trust of the participants grows with time.

Some people who live and work in a very conventional environment are worried that their acquaintances and colleagues would think them ready for the madhouse if they heard about their participation in a Reiki seminar. Since there are still many people who are quite confined in their way of thinking, this idea is not all that far-fetched. But in the practice this problem is rather rare since all the participants have a common experience with Reiki and, in addition, no one needs to tell anyone else where he spent the weekend.

I think it's too bad that many institutions, such as the churches, still make outlandish assumptions about Reiki. But there are also pleasant surprises. A man who had just become a Reiki channel was approached in turn by two colleagues who had seen how he put his hands on his belly after a meal and asked if he had perhaps participated in a Reiki seminar. Both of them had also received the First Degree some time back and were naturally quite pleased about the new Reiki colleague.

Sometimes there are also fears that the Reiki power comes from a demon or could bring disharmonious changes for the initiated and the people whom he treats. These fears quickly become irrelevant after some practice with Reiki. Those who experience the energy and its effects with a wide-awake consciousness convince themselves of it. Talking does no good here. It only causes more aversion since an insecure person then wants to protect himself, which is completely understandable.

Everyone bears the fear of the unknown within himself. When a person is confronted with an unfamiliar situation which cannot be explained, these deep-rooted feelings awaken. If this is how you feel, get involved in a few trial Reiki sessions. Get to know the respective Master beforehand in a personal conversation, phone call, or at a lecture in order to get a feeling for his energy. Talk to other people who have been initiated by the Master, if this is possible. What is said is not so important—gossip can even be encountered in the Reiki scene. Be aware of the mood between the lines, feel your way into it, and ask your intuition and not your head whether it feels alright with the idea.

You will only need a First Degree initiation once in your life. Make it into a celebration for yourself and find the security you need in order to open up to it. This is your responsibility. You will in any case become a Reiki channel through the traditional initiations during a seminar. However, you are the one to decide whether the time is already half over before you can open up and enjoy it or whether you have already found your standpoint to a large extent in advance. In the latter case, from the first moment to the last the First Degree seminar will be a sumptuous, sensory, serious, cheerful celebration which you will never forget.

Preparation for First Degree Reiki

During the registration conversation, the question arises time and again as to whether it is important to browse through Reiki literature, do certain exercises, fast, meditate, live in sexual abstinence, and so forth, before the seminar. It is naturally up to each individual to do whatever he feels could be important personally. However, with respect to the First Degree seminar, this is not necessary. The initiations also function if you have lived just from beer, pickled pork knuckles, and dumplings for the past ten days. With such a strain on the body, it is certain that you will not be aware of much that is happening there, but the initiation will always work!

However, I think it is better for each participant to be clear about certain things in advance and make it possible for his body to become more sensitive through a diet that places less strain on it. The more you can perceive and the more conscious you are, the more such a seminar will be touch you. The energy of the initiations effect a leap forward in the personal development of every person, in addition to opening up to the universal life energy. The intensity of this leap can be influenced by consciously opening up to Reiki and through the perception of the currently relevant personal learning processes. When I came to understand this course of events, I began sending each participant an information sheet before the seminar in order to make him aware of this as well. I am including the text here for you as well. In my opinion, it is also useful for Second and Third Degree initiations.

Take a look at it and make use of what you find appropriate for yourself.

"The participation in a traditional Reiki seminar always means an enormous leap forward in your personal development. The life energy processes introduced by the initiations and the intensive contact with the universal life energy will open new opportunities of experience for you and give you better access to the loving, living portions of your personality. Dormant talents can be activated and abilities that you already live can be expanded. You alone can decide how profound this gentle process of evolution will be for you!

In the days before the seminar, take some time for yourself on a regular basis and make it clear to yourself what you expect from your life, to what extent you have put these expectations into practice, and what you would like to open yourself for in the future. Do you desire more love and fulfillment in your relationships, would you finally like to have a satisfying occupational perspective for yourself, or would you like to solve a health problem?

Whatever it may be, the energy of the initiations and Reiki sessions during the seminar can introduce a positive development in every respect important for you. This means that you will not be healed in the medical sense of the word when you participate. But it can accelerate the developmental and learning processes within you, thereby contributing to a happier and healthier life in a comprehensive sense. Expect everything and nothing! Make yourself free for everything that will happen. Don't subject yourself to any limitations for your growth, and do open the door of your consciousness for the wishes concealed deep within your heart.

Let me say this quite clearly once again: The process that I have just described has nothing to do with your opening up for the universal life energy through the traditional initiations. You will become a Reiki channel in any case if you are initiated by a Reiki Master. You must do nothing and need to do nothing more than simply be there for this purpose.

Don't plan any scheduled or strenuous activities during the seminar days. Permit yourself to be there for yourself. The initiations can trigger deep processes of becoming conscious, and it is good to have the time to also work through them. You can come into an intensive contact with yourself—take advantage of this opportunity! For these reasons, you should also do without alcohol, nicotine, or other drugs during the seminar time. They decrease the ability to perceive and thereby your possibilities of consciously experiencing the coming changes."

So much for the preparation text. Before I get down to business in the next chapter, I would like to discuss one point which is addressed time and again, particularly with regard to the First Degree: Money!

Reiki and Money

"Why does Reiki have to be so expensive?!", "God's energy should be available for free, you shouldn't be allowed to make a business out of it!", "I think it's outrageous to take so much money for something that everyone is actually entitled to!", "That's a lot of money. You probably plan on being a millionaire within a year's time!".

These sentences are a small excerpt from the comments of people who had just heard of the course fees for the First Degree, Second Degree, and the Master Degree. Perhaps you have a similar feeling of indignation or lack of understanding. This is how I see the topic of "money and Reiki": When you buy a freezer that will last for perhaps five or six years, you place something like $500 on the counter. It would probably never occur to you have a discussion with the store owner on whether it is socially conscious to take so much money for a device that everyone could well use.

You know that he and many other people have contributed with their work, their personal efforts and experiences, their time, and by taking financial risks so that you can buy a complicated device like a freezer simply and relatively cheaply. Many people and their families live from this and put the money that they have earned back into circulation in order to acquire the other goods and services they need to manage their lives. If the store owner were to sell his goods with a 50% discount or even give them away, his family would go hungry and you would no longer have the opportunity of buying a freezer when you need one.

Perhaps you are now indignant and think: "How can he compare Reiki with a freezer!". Reiki power is naturally something different from a machine. But both need the personal dedication, the strenuously learned abilities, the time and exertion of people in order to be procured. On the one hand, the course fees are there to pay the seminar leader for his efforts. On the other hand, they represent the exchange energy of the Reiki student who receives what is basically an invaluable service in return. If the student doesn't give a return service or if it is too small, situations will occur similar to what Dr.Usui experienced in the beggar's quarter where he worked for a while. For $100 today you may get a half-decent cassette recorder or the First Degree. For $500 you can take a week's vacation or participate in a Second Degree seminar. For $10,000 you can become a Reiki Master (perhaps— it doesn't just depend on the money!) or, if you consider it more important, you can buy a small car. How much money is your contact to the universal life energy worth? Is it worth more or less than you spend on profane consumer articles?

Why should a Reiki Master give his time and not have the claim to a corresponding return service for his efforts? How can a tree grow, provide shade, create oxygen, bear fruit, and feed other beings without water, carbon dioxide, and nutrients? Have you ever seen a plant that voluntarily propagated "zero growth"? It is easy to spend money. There are so many beautiful things that we would love to have. If we cannot afford them all at one time, the thought often occurs that they should without cost. Yet, in the limitation of our possibilities lies an important source of help: We must decide and take into consideration what is most important to us at this time. Reiki is not absolutely necessary for every person.

You can be happy and healthy without Reiki. You can become enlightened and help other people find the way without Reiki. Don't believe there is any one thing that you are entirely dependent on in order to lead a meaningful, beautiful life. If you would like to have Reiki in your life, that's fine. But then you should also give the person who lovingly and responsibly stands at your side an appropriate compensation for the energy (it doesn't always have to be money).

Because of these reasons, it is not necessary to initiate welfare recipients or the unemployed for free or at reduced rates into a Reiki Degree. Saving up for a vacation or a new television set is completely normal. Why not save up for a Reiki Degree? If you feel the desire to become a Reiki channel, make it clear to yourself that this ability is a gift for which you could never pay. The Reiki Master who initiated you does everything he can in order to give you access to the energy and help you deal with it and its effects. The Master will also stand by you after the seminar if you have questions and has made an effort to acquire the abilities necessary to help you.

If this work is worth little or nothing to you, then attend a seminar on some other topic with a value that you can accept for yourself. If you participate in a Reiki seminar and are not convinced of its value, then you are deceiving yourself. Be honest and act without compromise. This will take you a big step forward, no matter what your decision is. A Reiki Degree should never be something that you "just take along with you."

These should be enough thought-provoking impulses for a start. There is certainly much more to be said on this topic, but I think it's better to integrate this continuing line of thought into the next chapter on the Reiki Degrees so that the ideas don't become too abstract.

By now you are certainly curious about what the First Degree involves. Whatever part of the Reiki path opens up for you with the initiations and what is the best you can make of it for yourself are the topics of the following chapter. Turn the page and look at the first step towards Reiki, the path of healing love.

Chapter Three

First Degree Reiki

In order to work with Reiki energy, it is absolutely necessary to receive the four initiations in the First Degree from a Reiki Master. There are various types of seminars for this purpose, which I will briefly introduce here so that you know what to expect in case you have not yet received an initiation.

If you are already a Reiki channel, then just skip this section of the chapter or skim through it to see all the possibilities of being introduced to the Usui System of Reiki. You may perhaps not be familiar with one or the other.

The Seminar

There are various ways of presenting the First Degree seminar. It can be carried out on one evening and two further days or on two days as a weekend seminar. If the seminar is organized as an evening course during the week, four consecutive evenings should be planned. If it is a vacation course, it can also last three or four full days. The course should never be held on just one day with all four initiations since each participant absolutely needs the time to experience the processes triggered through the contact with the universal life energy. Following the seminar, there is a period of three to six weeks in which important growth processes take place for each initiate. The body also frequently purifies itself on all levels during this time. Be attentive to yourself during this phase. Peace and quiet promotes the process of becoming conscious.

For these reasons, I don't think much of Second Degree initiations that take place either directly after the First Degree seminar or at an interval of two or three weeks later. The initiation naturally also "works" in these cases, but the developmental processes related to the emotions and the character don't get the full attention they need. Growth needs time. A lot and fast does not necessarily mean more in respect to the blossoming of your soul.

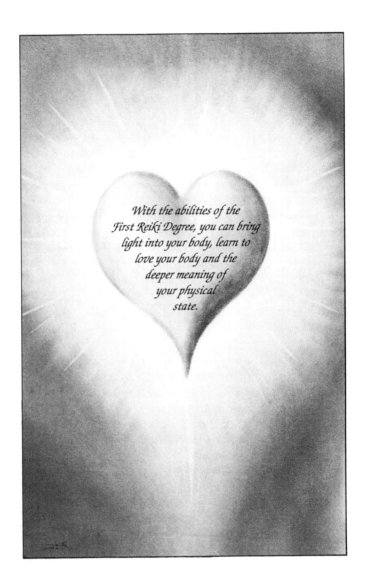

*With the abilities of the
First Reiki Degree, you can bring
light into your body, learn to
love your body and the
deeper meaning of
your physical
state.*

The First Degree seminar is designed differently by each Reiki Master. Although certain components, such as the four initiations, the telling of the Reiki story, and the instructions on a form of whole-body treatment and other techniques for applying Reiki are always the same, everything else is planned in accordance with the personality and interests of the respective Master.

This type of seminar design also contributes to keeping the course lively and exciting. Rigid concepts hinder the spontaneity of the seminar leader and that of the participants as well. The seminars held by the same Master often vary from each other in their structure. We constantly change ourselves, including the focal points of our interests. Responding to this liveliness very well suits the quality of Reiki energy, which does have an individual effect.

During my First Degree seminars, which usually take place from Friday evening to Sunday afternoon, I have observed similar behavior among the course participants time and again: The mood is very mental and skeptical on Friday. Critical questions are asked and the people involved respond with a great deal of reserve.

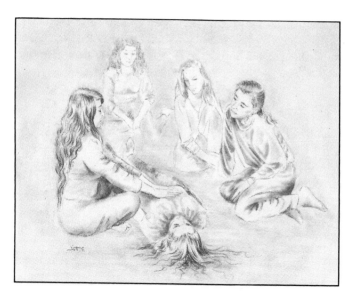

Scene from a Reiki seminar on the First Degree

After the First initiation, people are confused, deeply moved, and suddenly much more in tune with their feelings. The first contacts are made between those attending the seminar, Reiki treatments or feelings about experiences during the initiations are exchanged, and the atmosphere becomes more contemplative.

At the close of the session, I advise the participants to take a lukewarm shower before they go to sleep at the end of every seminar day in order to wash away the dissolved disharmonious energies from the aura; drink clear water, if possible without carbon dioxide in order to promote the life processes stimulated by Reiki; and, if possible, drink no alcohol in order to not impede the sense of perception. A diet that tends towards vegetarian fresh fruits and vegetables during the seminar time can also support the new orientation of the physical and emotional/mental/spiritual structures in some cases, but it is not absolutely necessary.

On Saturday, everyone is quite attentive and enthusiastic. Personal questions arise, and trust has already grown. After the further initiations, the atmosphere becomes increasingly relaxed. Towards evening, everyone is like one big, loving, and lively family.

There is almost a party mood on Sunday. The participants are very cheerful, and even those who usually have difficulties with closeness and loving contact can open up. At the close, they feel like they have been friends for years. Many deep friendships actually are created during the First Degree seminars. The question that is most often asked during the course is:

What Happens During the Initiations?

"Why is there such a secret about it? Why should I keep my eyes closed? What are you actually doing with me?"

I find these questions quite understandable. No one can expect that a person with closed eyes permits a ritual producing such enormous changes like the Reiki initiation to happen to himself without having some questions on the tip of the tongue. Yes— what happens in the initiations and why should the eyes remain closed? During the initiations, a Reiki Master uses the symbols and mantras (holy words that activate and direct certain energies) that Dr.Usui found in the old scrolls on Buddha's methods of healing. Through initiation as a Master and the symbols and mantras given to him, the Master is qualified to create a lasting connection to the source of the universal life energy for each individual.

In addition to the signs and words, there are specific rituals necessary for directing the energy into certain areas of the body that are involved in the channeling of the Reiki power. However, all these techniques are absolutely useless and do not function at all if the person doing them has not received the Master initiation in the traditional manner. Imagine the analogy of a radio—it doesn't work without electricity. For this reason, it was also not possible for Dr. Usui to work with Reiki after he initially found the scrolls. He is certain to have tried it. Only after fasting and meditating for three weeks—and with the grace of God—did he receive access to the source of universal life energy, without which all of the techniques cannot be applied.

Four initiations are necessary for the First Degree. Each of them has a different function. If all the initiations are not given on consecutive days, which means a maximum of four, the Reiki force does not remain and protection from outside energies is also not effective.

The effect of the Reiki initiations only affects the chakras indirectly. On a very deep energetic level, in the area of racial karma, it dissolves fixations of guilt which keep people from having direct contact to the universal life energy. This is why, with the exception of attaining the Reiki abilities which I will discuss later, the emotional/mental/spiritual effects of the initiations are different for each individual.

Although certain chakras are touched by the mental preparations, they are used more or less as doors. But the true changes take place on levels that are much deeper.

Why Should You Close Your Eyes?

Each person only needs to receive the initiations into a Reiki Degree once in his life. During the rituals, extensive harmonization processes take place within him. If he closes his eyes and feels within himself, he can consciously participate in this unique process. If he instead follows the Reiki Master's movements, that are obscure for him in any case, and constantly ponders on what effect this or that movement probably has, then he is not with himself and will hardly perceive anything of the fantastic things taking place inside of himself. It is therefore in the interest of those who are being initiated to close their eyes. In addition, the Master carrying out the ritual can naturally work undisturbed and more concentrated if six or eight pairs of eyes are not spellbound as they watch his movements.

Why is the Initiation Ritual Secret?

If no one other than the initiated Reiki Master can make anything of the ritual, then why must it remain so secret?

The reason for me is solely because of my respect for the source of Reiki power. I wouldn't like to have some people try out the course of the initiation, possibly in scientific mass experiments or as a pseudo-magical ritual, because they hope it could possibly work that way. The initiation ceremonies are something holy for me. I wouldn't want someone fiddling around with them needlessly. I feel that Reiki is too important for something like that. A further question that is frequently asked is:

Which Powers are Imparted By the First Degree Initiation?

There are essentially five different abilities:

1. The initiate becomes a channel for Reiki. He can bring this power down to earth at any time and pass it on with his hands when it is required. To do this, he does not need to concentrate, carry out certain exercises, or restrict how he organizes his life. If Reiki is needed, it is enough to lay on the hands or have contact to the recipient through the aura in order to let the power flow.

2. A type of protection is created to prevent the personal energy of the Reiki channel from being unconsciously transmitted to the recipient. This prevents a weakening of the person giving treatment and protects him from being confronted with the disharmonious structures of the other person on the energetic level. If this protection does not exist, it can happen that some of the energy of the person giving the treatment can penetrate into the inner energy system of the recipient and remain there.

3. The Reiki channel receives protection that prevents disharmonious energies from being transmitted to him by the person being treated. In this manner, the person who gives treatments remains free of sympathy afflictions and seriously disturbing external energies.

4. The sensibility for subtle energies is increased. After the First Degree seminar, many people notice completely new perceptions in their hands when they place them somewhere for a longer period of time.

5. All of these abilities are deeply anchored in the personality of the initiate forever. They cannot be removed by anything because they are ultimately a divine gift.

For this reason, each person only needs to participate in the preparatory rituals once in his lifetime. Everyone who takes part in the initiations of the First Degree course receives these abilities. There are no failed initiations as long as they are carried out by a traditionally trained Master with the symbols, mantras, and rituals that have been handed down. This may sound a bit presumptuous for your ears. After all, everyone makes mistakes. Why not Reiki Masters as well! But it is not the Master who ultimately carries out the initiation. He only produces the contact to the source of universal life energy and serves as a channel for the power. Everything else is effected from "above."

The things that human beings do are faulty and transitory. However, a bond created by God is not subject to the laws of the material world.

How Personal Growth is
Stimulated by Reiki

Something else occurs during the contact with the universal life energy, if the respective person is inwardly prepared to let it to happen. This is not a special ability, yet it can lastingly change a person's life: the opening of the heart. Here is one example of this: Before I came to the First Degree, it was very difficult for me to embrace other people. In the therapy group I participated in, if someone was sad I would think about whether it would be right to comfort him until the situation was over. I was afraid of closeness. Two days after the First Degree, I was once again in such a situation and spontaneously put my arms around my neighbor. Afterwards, I was surprised at my spontaneous reaction. I had not consciously prepared myself for it. Everything happened in a simple and natural way. Since then, I have frequently observed a similar normalization of behavior in other people after they participated in a First Degree course.

Deep-reaching changes take place in people through contact with the universal life energy. The divine spark within them receives a constant contact to the great divine light outside of us through the initiations. Each time when Reiki is put to use, it streams through the top of a person's head to his heart; from there it is directed to the hands. In the process, the heart center always absorbs some of the Reiki power which it transmits. The more a person permits his attention to dwell there, the more the heart chakra has the opportunity of developing. The energy flows more easily to the place where consciousness is. The many personal changes after a Reiki seminar result from this development.

The heart center organizes the energy of unity on all the physical and emotional, spiritual, and mental levels, thereby helping dissolve fears and promoting the efforts to let the mind and feelings work together. It is important for you to really understand this point. It opens up the working mechanism of Reiki on the spiritual, mental, and personal level: Reiki supports the development of a person in the direction of love, freedom from anxiety, truth, and perception, but it does not automatically produce this in the same manner as the five abilities described above, which are always imparted by the initiations of the First Degree.

Whether a person wants to take the path to the light with Reiki is also dependent on his free will. He must be interested in this path, with his attention directed to his heart in both the physical and the figurative sense in order to initiate and maintain the development. Every effort directed at the heart is then enormously intensified by the Reiki force. This process works like a sort of cosmic lever law.

Mikao Usui perceived the correlations in the effects after his experiences in the beggar's quarter and therefore established the five principles of life. Each of them touches on the aspect of unity, of love, in one of the five main chakras:

> *root chakra*—energy of aggression
> (don't get angry—just for today!)
> *sexual chakra*—energy of joy in life
> (don't worry—just for today!)
> *solar plexus chakra*—creative energy
> (earn your daily bread honestly!)
> *throat chakra*—energy of self-expression
> (try to be kind to all living beings around you)
> *forehead chakra*—energy of perception
> (be thankful for the many blessings!).

In this list, the *heart chakra* is left out or is addressed by all the five principles since the center of unity-promoting power of love is found there. (More detailed information about the chakras and their functions can be found in the appendix.) The Reiki life principles are a necessary supplement to the Reiki energy for mental and spiritual growth. When you become involved with them, gather experiences with your attitude towards the contents, and make the effort to gain access to their messages, you focus your attention on all your physical and spiritual levels with the power of love. This is the prerequisite for also coming closer to the light on the mental and spiritual level through regular Reiki treatments.

But there is one thing you should absolutely not do: slavishly follow the life principles. Drill has nothing to do with love. When you are angry, you cannot simply turn off your anger. The feelings are there and you should solely use your mind to make it possible for them to find an appropriate expression and express them in a manner that supports both harmony and life. As an example: When you are angry at a colleague, then scream out your anger on the drive home in the car and pound pillows against the wall. Feelings must have a possibility of physical expression, otherwise the firmly held energies form an obstructing armor of tense muscles with time. The cause for your feelings always lies within yourself. Another person triggers them within you. But he can only trigger what is already there. These are your energies. Live them out and make no one else responsible for them. Become concerned with the sense of the life principles, feel your way into them, and give yourself Reiki on a regular basis. Everything else happens automatically as long as you don't put a strait jacket on your feelings that prevents your lively growth.

Here is a summary of the above: Reiki treatments on a regular basis activate your self-healing and self-purification powers on the physical level. If you would like your mental and spiritual structures to also be stimulated to heal, then concern yourself with the five life principles and similar ideas in order to direct your attention in a way that promotes growth. Reiki sessions on a regular basis will support your efforts.

Practical Work with the Reiki Life Principles

Perhaps your response is similar to mine when I first saw the life principles. I had no idea how I should become involved with them. With time, I then became acquainted with some methods that made it easier for me to open up to them. Here is a particularly simple and effective way for you to work with all the principles:

Take one of the sentences. Read the text out loud. Listen to the sound of your words. Sense what is going on inside of you and observe the feelings triggered by the words. Don't censor them. Just observe them. In your mind, sit down next to yourself and watch how your spirit takes a position on the life principle. Is it agitated about it, does it find it funny, or does it explain exactly why it is impracticable? When you have listened to yourself for a while and noticed that nothing new is coming anymore, take a piece of paper and write everything down. Do this again without censorship, just as it came into your head. Now you have established the actual condition for yourself.

If you were honest with yourself, you now know to what extent you can accept this life principle. You can naturally also lie to yourself and say that you can manage wonderfully well with it and the practical translation of this sentence already takes place every day of your life. If this is the case, then turn over and go back to sleep! There isn't a human being who can perfectly follow this principle at every moment. This is not the meaning at all.

With its growth, a tree strives to reach the sun. It will never reach it here on earth because the tree will die before it succeeds. The situation is the same with the Reiki life principles. Make it clear to yourself that things will never progress to the point that you have truly integrated them into your personality. The path is the goal! The only way for you to make them applicable in a practical way is to become involved with their purpose, collect experiences by using them when it is possible for you to do so, and become conscious of your respective standpoint with regard to the principles. Just like Reiki, the five sentences should not become a prison for your feelings but help your consciousness to become more free. This can only happen when you recognize and learn to love your inaccessibilities, become aware of your emotional state as often as possible, and not try to talk yourself into thinking you are perfect or could ever become so here on earth. In addition to this general exercise, there are also some special "training methods" for each of the five life principles.

Exercises for the Individual Principles

Don't get angry—just for today!

Take this sentence as your motto of the day and try to not feel annoyed or angry. If you feel the anger rising within you, say to yourself: "I'm not angry!". Then feel within yourself to see how you respond to these instructions. When you do this, be honest and don't cheat. Otherwise, the whole thing will turn into a farce. A normal reaction to this "prohibition of anger" is that you will eventually become angry about not being permitted to become annoyed. Or that you suppress the annoyance and let other people have it through "justified critical statements" which injure them but leave you the possibility of playing hide-and-seek with your aggressions because you can prove to have a good reason for an apparently realistic reprimand.

I call this ploy the "manager method" because it is practiced so readily in the business world. If you have a very strong will, you can suppress your anger even longer, perhaps even long enough for it to create organic symptoms in the form of abnormal blood pressure or stomach problems.

A very effective anger-evading technique that is particularly widespread in the esoteric scene is the "substitute war." You look for some type of "reactionaries," "dark powers," the "evil world government," "demons," or whatever beasts worthy of hating are creeping around in the underworld and begin a rhetorical battle with them by placing the blame for the worst things in the world on them, from the business crisis to the coming end of the world (which has been predicted by "reliable" prophets).

The conflict can naturally take a more concrete form if you believe you are threatened by the "dark powers" and must fight against them with prayer, meditations, and visualizations (or whatever else occurs to you) for your own good, but especially for the well-being of the world. Just look around a little in the esoteric scene and you will catch a glimpse of the most adventurous outgrowths of this suppression of aggression in all its most colorful varieties.

As long as you seek the disharmonious elements outside yourself and refuse to see them inside of you, you will be sure of creating some in the outside world with all the spiritual energies that are available to you. In accordance with the old spiritual law "as within, so without!" you will encounter all the more darkness the more you collect the unresolved disharmonious structures within you until you believe that you alone are defending the light in the world as presumably the last good Mohican.

But that's not how things are. This principle can't be lived! Or can it? How about the following suggestion: You take "*don't get angry—just for today*" as an occasion to become conscious about the triggers and causes of your aggravation. You have already taken the first step if you have tried out the suggestions of the last paragraph and discovered your own methods with which you suppress anger, project it, or remove it from your conscious mind in some other manner. Write down your modes of behavior and pay attention at the next opportunity to which ones are you use in which form. It can be quite suspenseful to observe yourself at this type of hide-and-seek game. You will recognize and (I hope) learn to love your tremendous creativity with which you keep your vest clean to the outside world. There is an enormous potential within you. If you become aware of it, recognize its strengths, and accept it as part of your self, you can also use it later for other purposes which are more harmonious. Perhaps you can also laugh about your evasive maneuvers with time. You can also laugh at a comedy on television. As soon as you have learned to do this, you will have conquered a big piece of freedom and ability to love. As a result, you will have less occasion to become angry...

You can gain one other important perception by examining why you become annoyed. Everyone gets upset each day about many, many things which have nothing to do with them directly and don't even effect them. But there must be something that gets their goat and causes them to make ironic comments or have other reactions of anger. Only in very few cases are the circumstances actually related to what triggered the anger.

There is something that hits the affected person at a sore spot, a place that he skillfully conceals from himself and others. If he is obviously confronted with it, his subconscious reacts with panic. "Now I absolutely have to show everyone that this doesn't belong to me at all! Otherwise, they would believe that I'm also like that, and no one would like me anymore!"

Your anger will decrease with every sore spot inside of you that you get to know and consciously accept as something worth protecting. Annoyance is an emergency reaction. Learn to accept yourself with your weaknesses and dark spots on the vest. Then you will have less difficulty living out "don't get angry— just for today!" You will discover an enormous amount of energy which had just gone up in smoke because of anger before. The path there is endlessly long, but it's worth the effort of growing towards the light. With every step towards love, it will become lighter inside of you.

One hand on the forehead (third eye), the other on the pubic bone (area of the first chakra)—see illustration.

"Don't worry—just for today!"

Just as aggravation blocks the energies of the root chakra, worry blocks the sexual chakra, which I would prefer to call the chakra of joy in life since joy and the ability to have a relationship on the physical level are organized here on all levels. There is a simple exercise to get the suppressed joyful energy flowing again: consciously laugh for about 15 minutes when worries are weighing you down.

At first this will probably appear quite senseless to you. "Why should I laugh when things aren't going well for me?" But try it! With time, your laugh will become more free and at the end of the exercise you will notice that some of the mental and spiritual structures within you have relaxed as well. You will once again

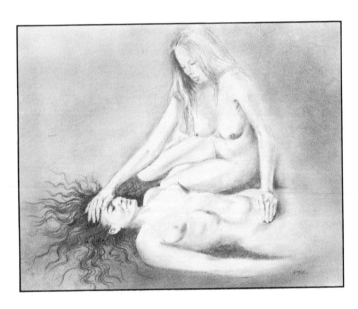

Balance of forehead and root chakra

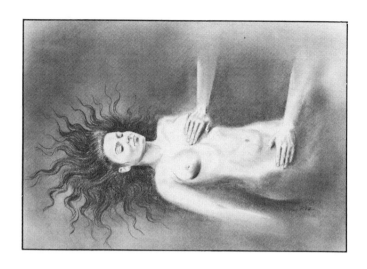

Balance of heart and root chakra

feel joy, the natural state of all living beings. Before and after this exercise, give yourself Reiki on the abdomen, the kidneys, the heart and solar plexus area, and the neck. It is thoroughly possible to laugh away health disorders, which are nothing other than a congestion in the flow of joy. Laughing is also good protection against the fear of black-magic influences. It is contagious. In a group of people who are connected by emotions, if someone laughs for a while the others will soon join in. Joy spreads and animates whatever was rigid. You can use this law to become more alive. You don't have to have a reason to laugh. Laugh just for the sake of laughing. This is meditative laughter. If you are not able to do this at the moment, then read comics or humorous books (see commented bibliography). Watch comedy films and get together with people with the intention of clowning around.

I have frequently noticed that I am much more open for Reiki when I permit myself to live out my cheerfulness. Don't confuse this type of laughter with laughing because of malicious glee. Although this variety can often be encountered, it is a harmful type of joy. Laughter and joy are the deepest human form of expressing thankfulness to our Creator. What can be more pleasing to God than when his children are joyful about the world created for them. The meaning of the principle *"Don't worry—just for today!"* is to demonstrate to you the power of joy and the life that it brings.

If you now say: "I can't be joyful, there are too many terrible and oppressive things in the world!," then try the following experiment: Take a day of vacation or, better yet, a weekend, and try to become aware of your worries. Picture all your worst fears as colorfully as possible: Your partner is unfaithful to you and abandons you. You lose your job and no one wants to hire you again. You don't get any unemployment money because getting fired was your fault. Friends and neighbors leave you and even refuse to greet you on the street. War comes, famine and reactor catastrophes, disease and the end of the world befall you. Nothing can stop these events! You are sentenced to boundless suffering and deserted by God and all the powers of good. How does this feel for you?

Feel within yourself and cry. If you can, lament and complain. Sense the agony and the rigidity that the worries in you are causing. With these fantasies, you are emotionally moving in the direction of death. This feeling spreads into your surrounding world because all feelings, not just the positive ones, are contagious. Be clear about these correlations! Then look out the window and perceive your environment. Is your situation really so catastrophic? Hardly! It is only your thoughts that are coloring the glasses of your senses—pink or gray. You decide how things should be. You decide whether you give off cheerful, animating vibrations or energies that can also cause paralysis in other people! If there really is a relevant occasion for worry, then go into that worry with all of your consciousness and bring all of your ideas about the catastrophe to the light. Cry and lament, let your fears and worries pour out of you. Afterwards, you will be free for the joy of life.

Silent sorrow brings sickness, but sorrow which is lived out is like a thorough housecleaning. At the end, pour out the rinse water and see how wonderfully everything now shines after the layer of dirt has been washed away. Like all feelings, you turn sorrow into poison when you suppress it. It will become the elixir of life when you accept it as an important part of yourself.

Special hand positions for this principle:

One hand on the heart chakra, the other just above the pubic bone (see illustration pg. 65).

"Earn your daily bread honestly!"

The practical experiences on this topic are very simple: During a workday, just examine in what areas you are dishonest with other people, as well as with yourself, as you carry out your job. You think that you're honest? Okay, let's take a look! How often do you work at something you have no desire to do but think it has to be done that way? How often do you do less than you could and still demand the same payment for it? How often do you give customers or colleagues an answer meant to have the effect of them believing that you are there for them when you really don't give a damn about their questions and needs? How do you act towards the Internal Revenue Service? Do you really declare everything you earn? How often do you cheat yourself by rendering a service for which you don't receive or demand an adequate return service? Can you really believe in everything you do or do you secretly judge your work to be damaging to the environment, human beings, or animals? The list could go on for quite a while, but I think you now understand what I mean.

This principle deals with the truth. With the exercises on the first two principles you already had the opportunity of training your love of truth in other areas. Now we're getting down to the nitty-gritty! The challenge is to "stop lying to yourself!" and "believe in what you do or change your life!"

This doesn't mean you should live a life of perfectly irreproachable conduct. This is humanly impossible in the long run since everyone defines morality in another way. But you can still make an effort and do your best in order to approach this goal as closely as possible. You could naturally also put your hands in your lap and do nothing at all. But when I really think about it, this is actually immoral as well. If you do nothing, you waste your talents that could help the world. Make it clear to yourself that you can never act without making mistakes. But make an effort to do so anyway and stand up for your errors. They belong to you, just like the rest. They are just as worthy as love as your

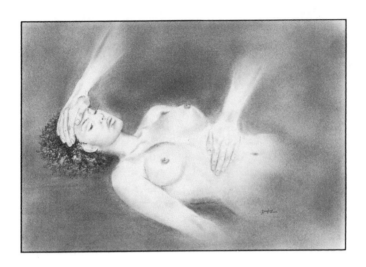

Balance of forehead and solar plexus chakra

perfect sides. A polished diamond is perfect in a certain sense, but it doesn't live like a human being! It cannot grow through its weaknesses and thereby recognize what love means. If order for this to be possible, the human being first had to be invented.

"Earn your daily bread honestly!" can help you let go of your claims to power if you admit to them. The Christian confession has a similar function. For a specific period of time, it can be an important experience for you to write down every night what you are ashamed of, when you have lied, when you have intentionally hurt someone or put them at a disadvantage, simply when you acted all too human. Look at it, even read it out loud, say the Lord's Prayer, and then burn the paper in the certainty that you will be immediately and completely released from all guilt when you do so. Later, it will be enough to do this exercise in your mind since it also has an effect in this manner if you are serious about it.

At some point you can stop doing this if you have understood the certainty of God's forgiveness. The rituals are for human beings, but God has already taken all guilt from you beforehand. By creating you, he has told the whole world that he wants you to be exactly like you are. You are good, beautiful, and worthy of love just like you are and nothing in the world can separate you from the source of love. When you let go of the conviction of being guilty, you open yourself up for love and therefore for healing on all levels. As long as you want to be guilty, a true healing is not possible.

Reiki hand positions for this principle:
Solar plexus and forehead (third eye) see illustrations pg. 68.

"Try to be kind to all living beings around you"

This life principle is based on experiences and the development of consciousness that you have gained by concerning yourself with the last principle. If you are more honest with yourself and stand up for your weaknesses, gradually learning
to love them, this progress will make it possible for you to be more loving with the living beings in your surrounding world since they reflect you in all your characteristic traits according to the law of "as within, so without!" It is very exciting to try out this principle in everyday life.

Try being very nice to the people you encounter for a few hours. Don't just do this when they are nice to you, but also completely without any preconditions and even when they behave quite miserably. You will be astonished how confused and uncertain your fellow human beings will react to this unusual social tone. Afterwards, use the first opportunity to write down the feelings you noticed within yourself. Do you feel good about your friendliness or do you feel uncertain and at the mercy of other people? Or do you perhaps feel even more certain than usual?

Then gather some experiences with the other extreme. Permit yourself to be really insufferable for a few hours. It is naturally important to find the appropriate surroundings for this exercise in advance. Otherwise, afterwards you may have to deal with the reactions of your fellow human beings who understandably did not find this game funny at all.

The best place for such games is in a self-realization group. It is a protected space in which you can try out how you feel with a new pattern of behavior within very wide limits. Everyone is there for you, and you do not need to worry about unpleasant consequences. Perhaps you know a few Reiki friends who would like to establish a self-realization group with you in order to learn to better cope with the life principles. Take the initiative and talk to them about it. You will create a fantastic learning opportunity for yourself and help other people grow at the same time.

A further possibility for training with this is writing down what you actually understand "being nice" and "not being nice" to mean. Do this as concretely as possible and then later go through the text with a good friend or your partner in life. Other people often understand this to mean something completely different. This will help you to relativize your perspective. Your glasses aren't the only ones through which the world is viewed. If your "fellow player" can also describe some situations to you in which he experienced you to be particularly nice or awful, you can receive even more important information on this topic.

One last tip: Start keeping a notebook and regularly writing down which words of kindness you would have liked to have said to someone or what you wanted to do for him. Take the next possible point in time to make this good and very consciously create an opportunity for this purpose. And what about the "unnice" wishes you have towards your fellow human beings that you cannot convey to them? Get yourself a punching ball and when you train with it paste on a picture of the dear fellow citizen to whom you would like to give your opinion. Afterwards, you will feel wonderfully relaxed and once again able to treat your neighbor in a truly nice and loving manner. Bawl him out when you are alone in your car or throw pillows against the wall at home and tell them everything you would have liked to have said to your "friend."

Even more possibilities for working off your frustrations without hurting other people are certain to occur to you—be creative! If you only bottle up your aggressions inside of you without living them out, everything will soon turn into a farce. If you like, take another look at the first life principle.

Reiki hand positions for this purpose:

Put one hand on the heart, the other in front of the throat; put one hand in front of the throat, the other at the nape of the neck or both hands as in the fifth head position of the whole-body treatment in the shape of a V in front of the throat; one hand in front

70

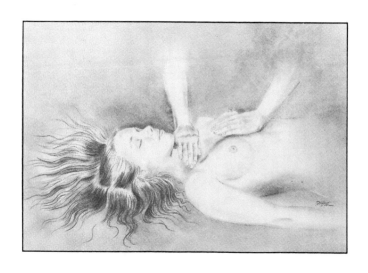

Balance of heart and throat chakra

of the throat, the other on the third eye; one hand in front of the throat, the other just above the pubic bone at the level of the second chakra. Put both hands to the sides of the balls on the big toes on the insides of the foot to the middle of the foot. (See illustration pg. 73)

"Be thankful for the many blessings!"

This is perhaps the most difficult principle. It requires no less of you than being thankful for everything you have, you receive, you are, you can learn, etc. The precondition for the first step into the practice with this principle are experiences and the development of consciousness with the first four principles. You now find yourself in the energy area of the third eye, and it is your learning task to let go of claims to power, instead developing trust and thankfulness. It is a matter of becoming conscious of your deep connection with all life. How does this work?

Let's start with the simplest thing. Make another list. This time write down all the things for which you can be thankful, meaning everything that isn't a matter of course for you. Include what you

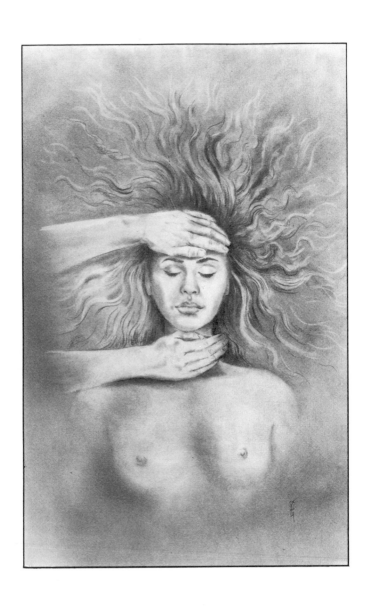

Balance of throat and forehead chakra

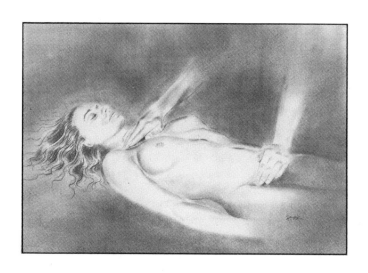

Balance of throat and root chakra

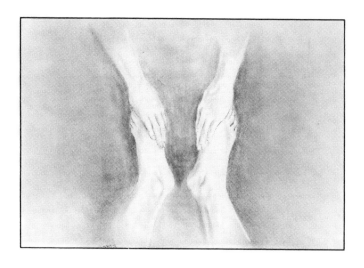

Harmonization of throat chakra through foot reflex zones

wouldn't have received without a bit of luck, what you have been given even though you didn't earn it, and what just "came to you."

After you have compiled the list, feel within yourself. Are you now truly thankful? Or are you asking yourself how one actually is thankful? You are already quite advanced when it comes to being thankful if you have now compiled the list mentioned above. The first step to doing this is becoming aware of everything you have been given by the world without having earned it yourself. If you then notice how much this really is (perhaps at some time you will also realize this is *everything*) and you think "hey, great, so many presents for me!," then you are thankful.

Please don't confuse gratitude with an exchange in accordance with the principle of return service. You have perhaps heard this statement at some point: "You could at least be a little bit thankful for this!". Here the other person meant to remind you that you are "indebted to him" and he could more easily have you do what he wants as a result. The sentence here absolutely doesn't have this meaning. When you follow the principle, it simply serves the purpose of doing something good for yourself and accelerating your growth. If you do the above-described exercise on a regular basis, you will notice in time that the universe, the World Soul, God, however you call him, her, or it, is there for you and upholds, feeds, and protects you. You only need to accept the things that are sent your way.

This principle is about developing the necessary basic trust for this purpose. The more you become aware of the presents the world has given you, the more secure you will become. If it is hard for you to see the presents—here are some examples: the air you breathe, the earth that holds you, the light of the sun, the rain, day and night, your dwelling, your friends, your daily bread, water, the money from which you pay your living costs: there are so many gifts for you!

But perhaps you sometimes feel like I do—I don't consider some things that come to me as a gift or don't want to have them, possibly thinking: "What should I do with this nonsense?" And that takes us to the next exercise.

Take time on a regular basis to write down the things you don't know what to do with. Perhaps you will already notice that this matter is leading up to the idea of a journal. This is actually the best way to make progress. It will help you get an overall

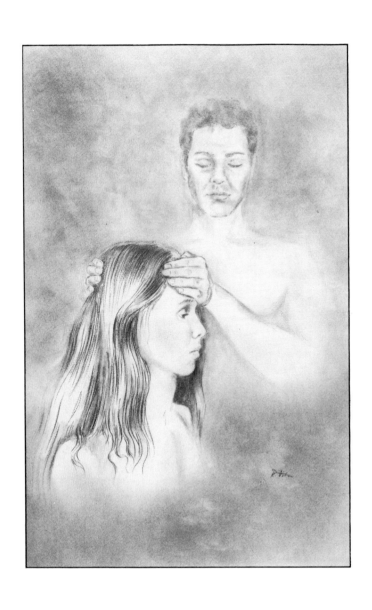

Specific chakra work on the forehead chakra

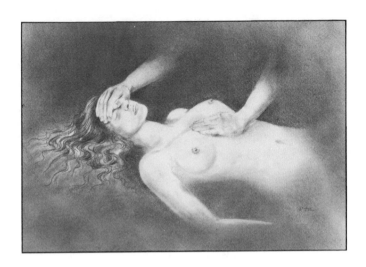

Balancing of forehead and heart chakra

view of your development and find the red thread of your life in time. If you know what is significant at the moment, it will be easier for you to become aware of how the universe has once again played an important ball into your hands. Oracle methods offer a further interesting opportunity for this purpose. I frequently like to work with the I Ching, but Tarot cards or runes are just as good. Using the pendulum is not suitable here, but numerology and astrology are applicable under certain conditions (both require a great deal of experience and expertise). Once again—learning to be thankful is not an exercise in submission but serves to expand your consciousness. It lets you open up for your path and the related assistance that the universe provides for you.

In closing, here is an exercise which can also be quite strenuous: If someone insults you, attacks you, talks about you in a derogatory manner, or hurts you in some other way, thank him for it! It will certainly be difficult for you, but you can gain much if you use this to gather experiences. In a quiet moment, sit down with your journal and write about the feelings you have become aware of in relation to this.

The purpose of this exercise goes very deep. On the spiritual level, those who love us the most are the ones who hurt us the most. Wait a moment before you continue to read. Let this sentence have its effect on you. Perhaps you could read it one more time. It is very important. Some paragraphs earlier I told you something about the mirroring function of your environment which helps you see aspects of your personality that you conceal at best from your fellow human beings and often even from yourself. It is only natural that precisely these are the things that hurt you the most when they are dragged into the public light. Learn to love your fellow human beings for this wonderful gift. Start by becoming aware of this function time and again when something hurts you. Then concern yourself with the sore spot within you. Become clear about its meaning and, if possible, its causes. Take yourself and your vulnerability seriously. From here, it is not much further to developing more love for your sore spots.

Here is an example of this: You meet a good friend and give him your hand—while doing so, you suddenly feel an intense pain in your lower arm. You have tendonitis. You will certainly not be angry with your friend because of it. It's not his fault that your arm hurts. In the near future, you will be careful with your arm, put a fixed dressing on it, and use a good remedy to heal it. If you are important to yourself, at the same time you will think about how your arm came to be afflicted. When you have figured this out, in the future you will probably be careful that this situation no longer occurs. Treat your emotional wounds in exactly the same way and you will be on the path to healing. I have also discovered that by concerning myself with my vulnerability the painful attacks from the outside lessened. Maybe you will have a similar experience.

Reiki hand positions and rituals for this principle:

Put one hand on the forehead (third eye), the other on the medulla at the back of the head. Put one hand on the third eye, the other on the heart.

The Reiki Meditation of Thankfulness

Here is a Reiki meditation on the theme of *thankfulness*: Sit down comfortably on a chair, the feet rest on the ground with the entire soles. Put the palms of your hands together in front of the heart. Your posture should be upright with the head resting on the neck. Now close your eyes and first direct your attention to your heart. Stay there until you have a good feeling for this part of the body, then direct your attention to your third eye. Now recite the Lord's Prayer. Say the words quietly and slowly or just think them. The effect is the same. Then say:

> *"Heavenly Father (or "Creative Force"), I thank you from my heart for all the blessings and gifts that you make available to me every day. I also thank you for everything that I overlook or consider to be insignificant because I do not understand its meaning. Please help me be open for your blessings and pass them on to other people according to your will."*
>
> *Now feel how you are breathing. Follow the way it goes in and out. It is breathing within you. Stay with your breath for a few minutes. Then stand up, lift your hands to your forehead, bow down, and say: "Thank you!".*
>
> *Let your hands sink down to your heart again. Keep feeling within yourself for another moment. Take a deep breath and open your eyes again.*

The exercise is now finished. You can also record this text on a cassette. This has the advantage that you don't have to memorize the words and the order, which is not important for the effect of this meditation. Concentration is a tensing of the senses. Here we are concerned with letting go and being attentive without the influence of the will.

In order to direct your attention, there is a simple trick. With one finger, tap lightly on the middle of your chest. Now clearly perceive this area. This is what is important. You can later do the same thing with the third eye in order to direct your consciousness there.

These are the last "training instructions" on Dr.Usui's life principles. Please do not subject yourself to the duty of coping with everything before you do the Second or Third Degree. An entire lifetime is not long enough to fathom and translate these five simple principles into action. I find it meaningful to have some thoughts of your own about the principles before you go to the Second Degree. Perhaps you can also begin to gather experiences with them in everyday life. Nothing more is necessary. Take your time. Rome wasn't built in a day either. The second principle *"Don't worry—just for today!"* should also tell you not to rack your brains about whether you are "mature" enough for something. The ripe fruits also fall from the branch on their own. Simply walk the path. Live Reiki-Do.

Stimulation for Development Offered by the Application of the First Degree Abilities

The methods of applying Reiki that you learn in the First Degree seminar can help you experience a great deal about yourself. The first of these is the whole-body treatment. Although this form of Reiki application is the most time-consuming, it is also the most intensive and holistic. It includes all areas of the body and ensures that they are addressed in a sequence that is meaningful for the energy of the body. The positions not only complement each other, but are also built upon each other. If you would like to know the details of this procedure, look them up in the *Reiki Handbook*. Everything is precisely described there. I would like to go into another aspect of this treatment method here.

Can you actually remember some occasion where you opened up to your body in a way that was similar to the whole-body treatment in its intensity and length? I had to answer this question with "no" for the time before my First Degree. It is not customary in our society for a person to occupy himself intensively with his body. Men are at an even greater disadvantage than women, who generally are more concerned with their bodies for cosmetic reasons. Except in the case of an acute illness, when you give yourself Reiki you open up to your body in a completely aimless manner. You become familiar with yourself from a whole new perspective, the physical and sensory. The whole-body treatment is one of the Tantric aspects of Reiki-Do.

With time, you will notice that every area of the body creates a different feeling of energy in your hands. You have an increasingly better and more differentiated feeling for your blocks and your openness, your reactions to the life-promoting Reiki power, from time to time. Perhaps you can quickly open up to these new dimensions of closeness with yourself, or perhaps it also initially triggers the deeply concealed fears within you that gradually rise into the realm of your perception. No matter how you react, you will attain a different, more holistic relationship with yourself.

In contrast to the meditative exercises or sport, you will learn to sensually open up to your own physical closeness. Hawayo Takata, the next to the last Reiki Grand Master, advised her students after the initiation into the First Degree to initially spend several weeks intensively giving themselves Reiki in order to get to know themselves in this new way.

During this time, writing a journal on a regular basis can be very helpful. Writing promotes reflection and the process of becoming conscious. The First Degree then initially leads you to contact with your own body, triggers the relaxation, purification, and self-healing processes within it, thereby creating new energies and the physical freedom for you to open up to the spiritual purification and growth processes.

It is possible for you to discover how difficult it is for you to be close to yourself at the moment. Perhaps because of your reluctance to give yourself Reiki on a regular basis and your desire to gladly receive it from others, you will notice this: You will be certain to also find excuses like "I don't have that much time for myself every day!". But you should have at least one to two hours time for your dog every day in order to play with it or go for walks. Your partner is certain to also need you for more than one hour a day, just like your children, if you have any. Are you worth less time? If you believe that Reiki is only important for the others, that you do quite well on your own, then think of the commandment: "Love your neighbor as yourself!" Both parties are expressly mentioned here.

Should you have difficulty in coping with closeness to yourself over a longer period of time, carefully examine to what extent this block hinders you. If it triggers more serious difficulties

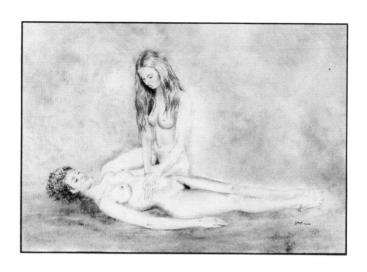

The First Degree—learning to accept the beauty of closeness.

in other areas of life or this structure bothers you, seek the help of a therapist you trust. Reiki will be a valuable aid in helping you work through your difficulties. After the experience of closeness with yourself comes the next step: At some point you will start giving Reiki to others.

Now you will become familiar with physical, sensory closeness to other people beyond erotic or athletic contacts. Before your Reiki initiation, when was the last time you quietly touched another person for more than an hour without any intentions? The intensive experience of closeness to others can in turn create more consciousness within yourself. Pay careful attention to your feelings when you do this. Take them seriously! Do this even if it means cancelling a session at some point or not going to a Reiki meeting because the closeness is too much for you at the moment. If you now allow yourself the distance that you need, you will more quickly be able to open up to closeness again. With time, closeness will have a completely different feeling for you.

Perhaps you will discover that your aggravation blows over and you become completely relaxed when you give Reiki. Or you learn to appreciate the beauty of quiet during the Reiki session and can finally open up to meditation. There is much to be discovered in the process—go for it!

There is an important experience you can also have with your partner. It frequently happens that partners do not like to give each other Reiki or claim that it doesn't flow when they exchange it. When they do a Reiki session with other friends, everything works quite well and they like it. Why is that? Reiki is always drawn in by the recipient. If an unconscious fear of closeness with the other person exists, no energy is drawn in and many possibilities of avoiding the contact arise under the influence of the unconscious mind. This constellation is present on the subconscious level for many couples.

If you notice these circumstances for yourself and your companion, definitely take the fear of closeness between the two of you seriously. Don't believe it just exists within the other person or within you. Relationships are not a one-way street! Talk openly with your partner about this problem structure. For a time, try giving each other Reiki briefly, but on a regular basis. Don't determine the length according to the clock. Each person feels into himself during the session. If he notices that feelings of reluctance are developing, he should immediately but calmly end the session.

If these difficulties continue, the two of you should clarify whether the fears of closeness also effect other areas of your relationship. If necessary, seek the help of a therapist. During a possible therapy, Reiki can help the two of you find each other more quickly and deeply.

A further dimension of closeness will open up for you when you meet with other Reiki friends and receive Reiki from the entire group. Try out this experience at least once and seriously confront the energies freed as a result. You can learn much about yourself in this process. Perhaps you will also have a completely different approach to this: You find it wonderful to be bathed in Reiki energy and consider it to be one of the "cream-puff" experiences in your life.

Closeness to yourself and others is then an essential theme of the First Degree. The more Reiki you give, the finer your perception of energy will become, allowing you to discover completely new impressions on the subtle level. Many people develop their sensitive talents in this way. Permit yourself this development as well! In time, you will learn to value it.

Giving Up Claims to Power

Before I give myself or another person Reiki for a longer period of time, I close my eyes for a moment, put my hands together in front of my chest as if in prayer, lift them to my forehead, and bow. Then I request, either quietly or in my mind, the permission to be a Reiki channel. This request and the exercise are absolutely unnecessary for the flow of the Reiki power, but they help me let go of claims to power and prepare for the session.

In doing so, I express my respect for the people to whom I will give Reiki. This is important to me in order to call to my conscious mind that he is no less worth loving, no less valuable and right than I am just because his weak points are more apparent than mine at the moment.

I don't know how you feel about it, but I think it's wonderful and impressive that Reiki flows through my hands whenever it is required to promote the life processes. The results are often immediately tangible and frequently also predictable. Even a short time ago, this caused me to frequently have the thought: "I just need to lay on the hands and then this and that will happen!". But it is not in my power to predict how the Reiki will work. I am "just" the Reiki channel.

The energy helps every individual to develop himself in the most suitable manner for himself. Even if I don't like his path. I should certainly still do my best to let Reiki flow to him. But I cannot and should not influence any further developments. With the bow and the request I call these circumstances into my conscious mind, and at some point it also becomes obvious to me that the course of the world is not dependent on my ideas. I find one last purpose of this exercise to be the development of thankfulness for the Reiki energy, which is always available to me when I need it.

No matter what I think, how I act, what I can do, or how I feel, God gives me the power. I thank him for this invaluable gift and am joyful about its life-promoting effects. Perhaps you will also see the sense of this little ritual. Then do yourself a favor and incorporate it into your way of handling Reiki. It will help you very much if you take it seriously. For others, it can be an important thought-provoking impulse when they notice your way of dealing with them and Reiki.

The Eternal Laws of Energy Exchange

A further significant experience for you comes with the conscious exchange of services and energies. During the First Degree seminar, you will hear that you should give some thought to what and how much you should request as a return service for longer Reiki sessions. This is not a matter of immediately holding out your hand every time you lay on hands for a few minutes to relieve a person's stress, for example. But when you give another person whole-body treatments on a regular basis, then think about what your time, your attention, and your individual effort is worth. Reiki power is free and available in unlimited quantities. Your lifetime is limited, and you must also perform the respective return services for your livelihood and your learning experiences. This all contributes to your general growth because every material service becomes much more valuable through the personal energy that becomes free during an exchange.

Here's an example: A painting by Dali has a material value of perhaps $150. Nevertheless, it is sold for many thousands of dollars and still not too expensive for the price. This is because the artist has combined the material components in such a manner that they make it possible for other people to have an expanded perspective of the world, possibly triggering deep processes of perception. This is naturally an extreme case, but it fundamentally applies to other value-creating situations. The material value is basically never paid, but the idea behind it and the personal creative energy are. The more unique the idea is, the more expensive the object becomes since many people could use this rare quality to complement their own personalities. If a service has been rendered and appropriately paid with a return service, a great deal of creative energy will flow in the ideal situation. Since every one of these energy qualities complements the recipient with an important element and thereby lifts his overall personality onto a higher level of development, every fair exchange of energy contributes to the growth of all participants.

But what is a fair exchange? I grappled with this question for quite a long time and found a conclusive answer for myself in a model derived from the chakra theory. In an optimal exchange of goods or services, as well as in another type of energy flow between various people, two levels should be touched on:

1. *The material level.* This means that an increase in material prosperity or the ability to create it must take place in this transaction. Material prosperity represents the roots of your life. If you are starving, you can neither learn nor love. You simply disappear from this plane of existence. A satisfactory situation on this level therefore represents the foundation for all the others.

2. *The emotional level.* This deals with the exchange of feelings. Closeness, warmth, love, joy, but also sadness or anger and related emotions, are required for every living creature to experience its life as meaningful on the deepest level. In terms of importance, this level comes right after the material one. A satisfactory exchange on this level helps the participants achieve a happier state of being. Through the exchange of feelings, human beings participate in the flow of life, which is the eternal process of growth and decay.

3. *The level of perception.* If a "transaction" results in an expanded state of consciousness for the participating partners, this process then contributes to opening up new perspectives of the Creation and making them accessible. A piece of consciousness has been added to the puzzle that we learn to put together in the course of our life. Perceiving means comprehending the correlations with the mind. Such a process can be triggered by reading this book, for example.

4. *The level of unity.* Here as well, when an exchange is completed both partners have created the perception of unity through the process of exchange. The fourth level can only be achieved when all the other levels have satisfactorily been taken into consideration as well.
It is difficult to explain this level, but easier to understand: Imagine you are standing in front of the altar with your beloved partner. The minister has just spoken the closing words of the ceremony. You look into your partner's eyes before the rings are exchanged. Now you feel it—this is what unity is like.

This model is naturally quite abstract. Let me explain the entire matter through an example within this context: You give Reiki to an acquaintance. In return, she invites you for a meal. Through your service, you have provided her with the ability to be more relaxed and therefore productive in her everyday life. She has saved you the effort of shopping, cooking, and serving the meal. The exchange here is on the first level (material). During the treatment, your acquaintance can increasingly let go and feels quite good because you are looking after her. The situation is similar when she cooks for you and you are properly taken care of. This is the second level (emotional). As a result of the treatment and her hospitality, you have both understood that it is better to live in a community in which each person is there for the other than being alone and lonely. Now you find yourselves on the third level (perception). Perhaps you feel closer in a mysterious way because of this process. Before the Reiki session and the subsequent invitation you were friendly acquaintances. Now you suddenly notice a deep familiarity and a wordless sense of agreement when you encounter each other. The makes both of you happy, and you enjoy being close to the other person. You have become friends. Now you have completed the exchange on the fourth level (unity) as well.

Play out this model with various situations with which you are familiar. It doesn't matter whether you consider a marriage or purchasing a pair of pants through these glasses, it always works. If you search around in your memory and look at some experiences under this aspect, you will discover that you were quite satisfied each time an exchange touched on at least three of these levels: "transactions" which touched less than two of these levels of exchange probably produced deep dissatisfaction within you. Afterwards, you most likely longed for a situation in which the neglected levels were touched as well in order to balance out the deficit.

Think of these experiences in future situations in which you exchange energy and be sure that as many levels as possible are affected. This is how you can consciously contribute to the growth of everyone involved. I find it quite suspenseful to occasionally write down which levels were touched on certain occasions. With time, this will strengthen your ability to achieve a better intuitive understanding of energy exchange. You will no longer cheat yourself by convincing yourself that because of some drearily moralistic reason you do not deserve to demand a return service for a service you have provided or consider another person to be bad when he asks for a return service for his efforts.

The Decision on the Second Degree

After about two or three months of experience with the First Degree, you can register for a Second Degree seminar. But you should really allow yourself this much time and not run from Master to Master to find one who will initiate you just one week later.

If you have not taken advantage of any or merely a few opportunities to use the Reiki power during the time of two or three months, you should give some hard thought to why you now want to do the Second Degree—do you plan not to apply it as well? Or would you just like to have one more certificate? Do you just want to be able to join in the conversation on the topic? Why? Be honest with yourself. You will possibly save a great deal of money in the process.

The Second Degree is something very beautiful, significant, and holy. You shouldn't do it "just to see what it's like." It is not intended for this purpose. The next chapter will describe why people do the Second Degree, the hopes and fears they connect with it, and which possibilities of personal growth it offers you. It will certainly be much different than you think. Or do you perhaps like to read from the back to the front (like I do) and already know everything? In this case, I wish you much enjoyment with the second chapter!

Summary

With the opportunities of First Degree Reiki you can learn to:
- create closeness with yourself
- allow closeness with other people
- understand the deeper meaning of relationships
- apply the five Reiki life principles and healing principles discover their deeper significance for the healing of your body and your spirit

- develop your sensitivity and thereby receive the possibility of perceiving the world in a more sensual and lively manner
- giving up claims to power
- basing your lifestyle on trust in a higher power
- experiencing unity
- understanding the eternal laws of energy exchange
- accepting and loving the understanding of the deeper meaning of health disorders and other weaknesses in your personality
- feeling God's presence
- accepting your emotions
- living love.

Some Instructional Sentences as an Approach to the First Degree

Always give Reiki when you have a desire to do so. Never give Reiki just because you believe you have to.

Try to perceive your own feelings as often as possible during a Reiki session.

Concern yourself with the five life principles, find your own viewpoint on them and experiment with them.

Every morning when you get up, say to yourself: "I do not live in this world in order to be perfect, but to learn to love by accepting my weaknesses!".

Allow yourself the consciously experienced closeness to yourself and others. Experiment with Reiki. Give free rein to your creativity. Working with Reiki can be a wonderful adventure for you.

Reiki releases tensions by letting the blocked energies flow once again. If you become fearful, sad, cheerful, or happy during a Reiki session, you will know what energies you have held onto. Then you can think about why you have done this and if you still tend to block this force when it becomes active.

If you give yourself Reiki on a regular basis, you will have the power to grow. You decide where and how this takes place on the mental and spiritual level by directing your attention to one area of your character.

Chapter Four

Second Degree Reiki

Why Do People Come to a Second Degree Seminar?

Registration for this seminar is often sparked by a particularly impressive experience with Reiki.

For me, this was the disappearance of a serious inflammation of the pelvic organs in my first wife, Manu. This happened practically overnight through a distance treatment by our Master Brigitte Müller. The day before, a blood sedimentation and physical examination had still shown the symptoms of a serious inflammation. The next day, a gynecologist was to refer Manuela to a hospital. However, as a result of the half-hour distance treatment the evening before, all subjective and objective signs of the illness had disappeared by the time of the doctor appointment and never appeared again. At that point, it was clear to us that we would participate in a Second Degree seminar.

Other people feel the strong desire to become more involved with Reiki than is possible through the contact treatment. Some individuals would like to advance their spiritual development through the initiation and the Second Degree techniques of mental treatment. Others are simply tremendously curious as to how and whether such distance healing really works.

One important reason for many therapists who work professionally with Reiki to come to the seminar is the enormous acceleration of the treatment and the possibility to effectively provide many people simultaneously with the universal life energy.

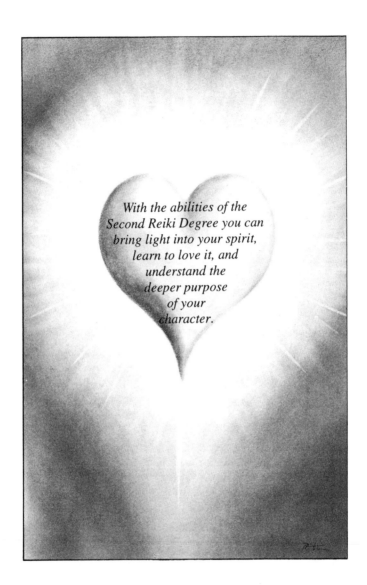

*With the abilities of the
Second Reiki Degree you can
bring light into your spirit,
learn to love it, and
understand the
deeper purpose
of your
character.*

The Fears

Since everyone who registers for the Second Degree seminar has already participated in a First Degree seminar, most of the fears have already been dispersed. However, the concern that there could still be a fraud involved in the Second Degree still remains since the few comments by the Reiki Master at the close of the First Degree seminar contain such unbelievable things that "healthy common sense" can no longer keep up. Which isn't necessary since Reiki does not work—thank God—through the rational mind.

Even more than in the First Degree, before the Second Degree the question is posed as to why the seminar has to be so expensive. I don't want to discuss the fundamental issue of service and service in return again, since it was treated extensively in the last two chapters. However, in my opinion it is important to give a special explanation of why the price is so much higher for the seminar, which is usually shorter in comparison to the First Degree.

The Second Reiki Degree contains an enormous range of possibilities for working with subtle energies. They are limited practically only by the bounds of your individual fantasy.

At the same time, this entails a great responsibility. When you receive an ability, it becomes a component of your personality from that time onwards. Seen from the viewpoint of cosmic laws, it is your task to become involved with it and collecting experiences.

Since we human beings basically take expensive things more seriously, one way to ensure that a person really makes use of the Second Degree is to put an expensive price tag on it. In addition, the high price causes the respective individual to give serious thought to whether he truly wants to participate in this seminar or if the better choice would be to take a vacation instead. This is really a matter of personal preference. It is not absolutely necessary to do the Second Degree. If you are more interested in something else, it would be better for you to occupy yourself with it instead. Stimulated by the stumbling block of "an expensive price," you can learn much about yourself. And this is free of charge, even before the seminar.

Summarized in brief: The price is meant to discourage all the people who do not take the Second Degree seriously or seriously enough. This method naturally also has its flaws, but I think it is the one best practiced in our society. Or would you like to first clean your Reiki Master's ashram for three to four years in silence before being admitted to the Second Degree?! If you have searched your soul and made the weighty (this is also what I mean!) decision to do the Second Reiki Degree, then you will participate together with a number of other people in a seminar with a Reiki Master who will initiate you and give you a precise explanation of the various fundamental possibilities presented by the Second Degree.

Yes, they are a present—when you have worked with the new possibilities for a while, you will understand why.

The Seminar

There are usually divided in three evening courses or weekend seminars with a minimum of one evening and one day to one evening and two full days, as well as vacation courses that run for a number of days. As in the First Degree, the seminar organization in terms of time and partially in relation to content is handled in quite different ways by the various Reiki Masters.

For the participants, this has the advantage that their Master also has a great deal of enjoyment during the course and can make the program lively and exciting. Boredom is always the result when a standard procedure is just reeled off.

During the seminar, each participant receives an initiation that firmly anchors the symbols and mantras of the Second Degree within him. At the same time, it makes sure that they are activated and therefore become useful for the participant. Without this energetic ritual, the signs and words have no effect. In contrast to the initiations of the First Degree, the emotional body— meaning the level of the feelings, fears, and hopes—is affected to a lesser extent. It is no longer necessary to bring the deep karmic layers of the personality into contact with the divine light since this connection already exists.

Now it is a matter of stripping away the disharmonious structures on the mental level which impede people in using their full potential of abilities created through this connection. Among other things, the third eye (the forehead chakra) is activated. This sparks better perceptive abilities in the subtle area, sometimes even spontaneous clairvoyance in some people, an intensification of the intuition, and more interest in self-realization and finding one's own path in life. The essential energetic changes then take place on the mental level in the Second Degree. I will give a more detailed explanation of this level and its tasks below.

The initiation is usually given towards the beginning of the course since it is not possible to work with the techniques without it. Next, the symbols and mantras are given to the participants, who learn them by heart. It takes several hours for all of these tools to be adopted for personal use.

Afterwards, the methods for putting them to proper use are imparted and then trained by the use of practical examples. You will already notice that this seminar is completely different than the course for the First Degree. During the introductory seminar, the intuitive feeling was involved the most, and now the head is the main focal point. Yes—and that's it for the Second Degree seminar. "That's all?" you think? I am firmly convinced that the Second Degree can effect more changes for an individual, as well as offer many more possibilities of applying the Reiki energy than the First Degree. Perhaps you will share this conviction after reading the next section, in which I will tell you about everything you can do with the Second Degree.

The Tools of the Second Degree Reiki

In order to not promote any false hopes: I will print neither symbols nor mantras here. There is no way for you to use them without initiations, and I consider them too valuable to reveal them in order to just satisfy curiosity.

The fundamental means of the Second Degree include:

1. Energy Intensification

This is one possibility of making more Reiki energy available than the maximum you can normally transmit on your own (energy intensification). The law of "the recipient determines how much and where he wants to absorb Reiki" is not repealed by this. In each application, the available Reiki energy is increased by 10 to 15 times*.

Since as many applications as desired can follow each other, there is theoretically no upward limit to the flow of Reiki energy. When you use this technique, the treatment times are reduced drastically for both the contact treatment and the distance treatment. In the contact treatment, the time can be reduced to about two minutes per position. In practice, an even shorter amount of time doesn't do the job since a certain amount of time to open up to being touched is simply necessary in direct physical contact. However, for a distance treatment with the Second Degree, a shortening of the time for a whole-body treatment of 10 to 20 minutes is completely realistic. In this case, the contact is purely subtle and energetic. In addition, the course of treatment differs considerably from the contact whole-body treatment so that the impact of the energy intensification should take full effect. In such a distance treatment, the effect can be much more intensive than for a 90-minute whole-body treatment with the means of the First Degree. Particularly for professionally active Reiki therapists this opens up new perspectives because an essential reason for a healing practitioner, for example, to not use more Reiki in the practice is the relatively extensive amount of time required. But even non-professionals can make good use of this technique. One example of this is when you give Reiki to yourself or your relatives. Food can be charged much more quickly with Reiki and gemstones (also see under "Reiki and Crystals" in *The Complete Reiki Handbook*, pg. 113) can be more easily and quickly cleaned energetically and charged with Reiki. In the same manner, cosmetics and drinking water can be purified within a short time period through the effects of Reiki power.

Summary: Everything that you can do with the First Degree can be done more quickly and intensively with the Second Degree technique because the boundaries of energy flow are suspended. This possibility is a consistent further development of the confrontation with the topic "time for yourself," which belongs to the personal learning experiences of the First Degree.

---

*This is just an estimate.

When these experiences have been essentially lived out and worked through during the time with the First Degree, it is no longer necessary for the purpose of personal development to spend as much time with the experience of closeness. You naturally can and should have time for closeness in the Reiki applications if you have the feeling that it is particularly important for you. But the automatic limitation caused by the restrictions on the intensity of the Reiki power no longer exists.

The Second Degree frees you from many limitations. And not just in respect to the treatment time!

2. Distance treatment

This is a technique with which you can reach, provide Reiki to, and exchange information with everything that lives (distance treatment). With this, you can basically establish a connection to everything in the world because, in the deeper sense, *nothing* is without animation on this level of existence. Everything was created from and by God, the source of all life!

In relation to Reiki, this method releases you from the limits of space and, as you will see below, also from the limits of time. You only need the name and a picture or a personal impression, such as the sound of the recipient's voice. You can, for example, comfortably sit in your armchair in your apartment in Hamburg while the friend who wants to receive Reiki camps in the Brazilian jungle. With the exception of the physical closeness, the energy transmission will be just as strong, and frequently even more effective, than if both of you were in the same room. A further possibility that this technique offers you is the simultaneous treatment of many people with Reiki. In the same period of time that you require for one distance treatment, you can provide 10, 20, 30, or more friends with abundant Reiki at the same time. This aspect of the possibilities of the Second Degree frees you from the limitations of spatial contact.

You are no longer dependent on the proximity of a person in order to give Reiki to him. This is also a suspension of limitations no longer necessary after living out the experiences of the First Degree. Before, the physical closeness and the opening up to physical contact with others was very important. The important thing now is to open up to the mental contact. When these opportunities for growth are used, it is no longer absolutely necessary to maintain the limitations. If they would continue to exist, it would not be possible to have truly new experiences. The experience of distant treatment also expands consciousness. Your mind cannot avoid perceiving that space is just an illusion in the deeper sense. You will experience that the restrictions you have considered insuperable up to now do not exist in reality. Think about the consequences that result from this, and you will come to the conclusion that science fiction does not just contain "fictions" or fairy-tales, but much more.

With one particular application of distance treatment, you can reach into the past or the future, if you want, and give Reiki directly or through the mental healing method in certain situations. It is therefore possible to give Reiki to a formative situation of your childhood and, as a result, harmonize its effects.

Were you ever seriously ill and still have a heavy burden to bear today because of the consequences? "Ah, yes," you think, "had I only been able to do back then what I can do now!" With the Second Degree, you can! Establish a contact with yourself when you were ill and send Reiki to yourself over a longer period of time. The effects are often unbelievable.

You can approach the future in the same way. You know that you will have to work long and intensively the next day. You're fine right now, but tomorrow...! Apply the Second Degree method in a certain manner and give yourself Reiki now so that it reaches you tomorrow at a certain time. Do you think I'm crazy? I can't prove it to you right now, but you can experience it yourself when you have the Second Degree or ask other people who have learned to work with the Second Degree in this way.

So, the restrictions of the passage of time have now fallen away as well. Could there be anything else? Oh, yes! When I told you above that you can reach everything with the distance treatment, I really meant it. Now there are many things that you could reach, but in which area could this be of interest to you? For example, I like to give Reiki to my Higher Self and my Inner Child. Sometimes I also do this for other people. Why?

In order to explain this to you, I must backtrack a bit. We all have three different parts (archetypical partial personalities) which are connected with us in the closest way possible on the one hand, but can also have completely independent modes of behavior and different functions and possibilities on the other hand.

Let's start with the conscious portion. It is also called the *Middle Self*. It can think, calculate, draw logical conclusions, consider why this or that has led to a certain result or will lead to that result. This is where all the information that reaches a person through the five "common" senses is evaluated both consciously and unconsciously.

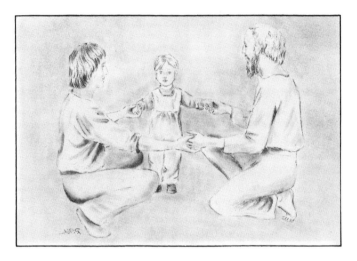

The union of the three parts of an individual's personality:
Higher Self—Middle Self—Inner Child

The *Middle Self* does not possess a memory or feelings. It has no extrasensory perceptions and no conscience (this is also associated with the memory since it is formed through experiences). The information that the *Middle Self* has evaluated is stored by the *Inner Child*. It is also the source of feelings. Here is where morality, ethics, and the conscience develop.

If excessive demands are placed on the Middle Self's ability to sort information, through too many important impressions perceived at the same time, for example, the Inner Child receives the information in an unorganized manner, and the Inner Child must sort it into the memory retention according to it's own possibilities. However, these do not include the ability of logical evaluation.

This is how many fears, feelings of guilt, and dogmatized concepts of morality arise. Such situations occur especially often during childhood since the Middle Self does not yet have as many possibilities of evaluating the information as an adult during this developmental period. It is quickly overtaxed at some point. For this reason, the roots of most psychological problem structures lie in childhood. Yet, at a later point in time, accidents, emotional shocks, or constant mental exertion can cause such unorganized memories to be collected. The instincts and the extrasensory perceptions are also at home in the Inner Child. Here too is the source of the personal energy at an individual's disposal, which can be used for all forms of magical work, among other things.

The personal life energy (Ki) is constantly replenished through food and the air we breathe. It is not identical with Reiki, the superpersonal, universal life energy. Through its extrasensory abilities like telepathy, the Inner Child can create a direct connection to the *Higher Self*. The Middle Self cannot do this. It is much too shaped by the logical, comprehensible structures to imagine such non-causal phenomenon and thereby relate them to the realm of the possible.

For this reason, "rationalists" have such difficulties when it comes to feelings, spiritual matters, and non-logical correlations. They do not accept their Inner Child, which means it cannot help them understand these manifestations. The Inner Child does not think logically like the Middle Self. Its way of looking at things and dealing with them is shaped by emotional energies, images, sounds, smells, stimuli, and symbols.

On this level, the correlations are created not through logical, but through non-causally determined similar features, such as synchronicity, or other sympathetic relationships. Since magic is also at home here, you will now perhaps understand why magic rituals are based on sympathetic correlations instead of logical ones. For example, think of the voodoo doll of black magic, as well as the chicken feathers and little healing poems used as magic formulas to cure warts and shingles.

The Inner Child is easy to impress with pomp, theatrical gestures, and the like. It likes to play and is curious. In general, it tries to help you, except when you have annoyed it. This can happen if you call it dumb, silly, or wicked. But if you take it seriously and help it to better understand the world, in addition to its very own manner of understanding, it will also learn the way of the Middle Self in time. And by becoming involved with your Inner Child, you will also get to know and love the childlike perspective of the world in addition to the sober-minded, logical manner that you have already mastered.

"Become like children!" said Jesus, meaning that it is very important for us to be friends with our Inner Child, to learn to love and respect it. The ability to use the pendulum also takes place through the Inner Child. The pendulum is a type of display instrument with which the impressions that the Inner Child receives through its subtle sensory organs are transmitted in terms understandable for the Middle Self. However, before the transmission, all this information goes through the filter of the Inner Child's fears, hopes, and feelings of guilt. This is why the pendulum is not necessarily suitable as an oracle, for orientation on the path of life, or for attaining information about spiritual correlations. Oracles such as the runes, I Ching, or Tarot are much better suited for these purposes. They are directly controlled through the respective Higher Self and therefore contain the right information and evaluation of correlations in the holistic sense.

The Higher Self is the divine aspect of the human being. It is familiar with the life plan chosen by an individual and knows about past lives. The Higher Self is not connected to time and space like the other two parts of the self. It likes to help them both in their development, when they expressly desire this and provide it with the energy the Higher Self needs to have an effect on the material level. This procedure is commonly called "praying."

You certainly know as well that not every prayer is answered. Why is that? In order to pass the Middle Self's prayer on to the Higher Self, the cooperation of the Inner Child is necessary. If this part considers itself to be too guilty, evil, or unworthy for a contact with God or considers the request to be "immoral" or not permissible, it will refuse the cooperation and not create the necessary connection. In the process, the Inner Child's appraisal is not based on logical correlations, but, as described above, oriented upon the learned moral concepts that have been assumed from the parents, for example. If it makes the connection without knowing how it should send energy to the Higher Self so that the latter can achieve the realization of the prayer, still nothing will come of it. "Pretty complicated!" you groan? I don't believe so. Let this information work within you for a while, then you will notice that it may be unaccustomed, but actually not complicated.

One example of these correlations is the ability of some faith healers. As long as they demand no money for their efforts, they can heal. Their Inner Child then believes that it is pure enough for the cosmic power. When such a healer asks for money despite this, the Inner Child finds this act to be immoral and not in accordance with the divine will. As a result, it does not dare request healing energy from the Higher Self. The faith healer can no longer heal until he has atoned his "offense" and once again continues without an exchange of energy. Other healers, who do not carry this moral structure within themselves, are very much able to accept larger sums of money for their services and bring about wonderful cases of healing at the same time. This is then completely a matter of the acquired character structure. Some people also call this karma.

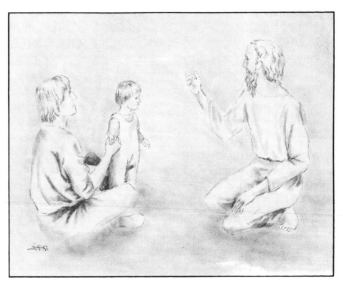

The Higher Self supports the Middle Self and the Inner Child in their growth processes, when they desire it.

Contact with the Higher Self is very important for you. It can help you properly cope with difficult situations in a holistic sense. You will more frequently come together with people and situations that are appropriate for you and can help you to learn what is important for you. Through regular contact with your Higher Self, you will receive the necessary security to steer your boat of life, and this will help you develop the personality portions of the Inner Child and the Middle Self. This development will increasingly tune your entire personality to the energetic level of the Higher Self:

This voluntary tuning is the actual sense of human life. On the customary paths, it is quite tedious and complicated to achieve true contact with the Higher Self. What many people who seek this connection experience is at most an intensive contact with the Inner Child and its colorful world of images. And this is quite fine since a person should first come into contact with himself before trying to establish contact with God. A tree first needs the connection to the earth if it wants to grow to the light.

On the Reiki path, the level of the Inner Child is essentially cleared with the possibilities of the First Degree. But later there will also be many opportunities to play and learn with it.

One feasible way of reaching the Higher Self by clarifying the relationships to the Inner Child and its feelings of guilt is the HUNA teaching according to Max F. Long (see Bibliography). I have adopted essential information for the understanding of Second Degree work from this teaching, which is based on practical experiences.

The HUNA theory fits in so well with Reiki practice that they are practically made for each other. In my opinion, both of them had a common origin far back in history. Be that as it may, you can achieve excellent results in any case if you use the Second Degree tools and at the same time take the HUNA perceptions into consideration.

By use of the Second Degree abilities, the Inner Child as well as the Higher Self can be reached directly. You can exchange information with both of them, suggest and discuss paths of co-operation, and mobilize energy through your Reiki abilities in order to make life easier for yourself and others.

When you come into contact with your Inner Child, the communication will initially take place through symbols, colors, pictures,

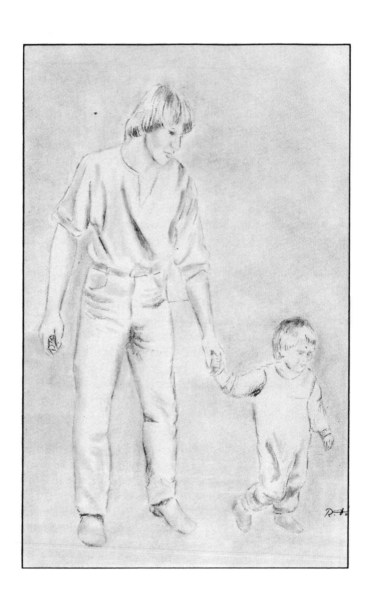

*When the Middle Self and the Inner Child of a person learn to
accept each other ...*

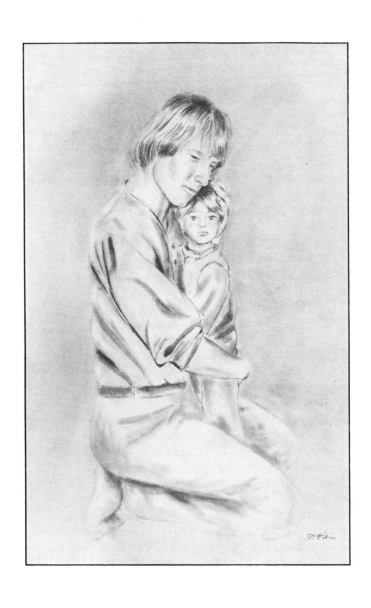

... they become a loving power team.

feelings, and the like. You cannot necessarily speak directly to your Inner Child with words. It is easy to impress, playful, likes to please, but also quickly peeved or bored if something goes against its grain. Explore your fears and hopes together with it, help it get a different perspective on the things that confuse it or create feelings of guilt within it, and let it help you become more playful and lively, follow your curiosity, and take your feelings seriously. With time, you will both get along better and give each other mutual support. Your Inner Child will give you much lively energy, which you can use in harmony with the terms of your Higher Self in order to properly arrange your life in the holistic sense.

When your Middle Self and your Inner Child learn to work together in the sense of karma, they are a real "power team"!

The Reiki contact with your Higher Self will be even more exotic than the preceding contact to your Inner Child.

During the first meditations with your Higher Self, you will probably receive less concrete impressions. Don't even expect this. Make yourself free for whatever happens. After each session, which should not exceed 10 minutes once a week at the beginning, you will be quite confused, disappointed, or even deeply impressed—without actually knowing why. Don't ponder about this. Let the contact happen time and again! In the course of time, both your body and your spirit will enter into a deep-reaching harmonious process of growth.

When you have noticed this process, you can go one step further. Give your Higher Self several minutes of Reiki and tell it that it can use this energy according to its own will. Ask your Higher Self for help in a matter that is important to you and which you would like to wisely settle in a holistic sense. Tell it that it is important to you that this matter be resolved in such a way that it does justice to all the participants (this is very important!). Afterwards, give it several minutes of Reiki again so that it can have an effect on the material level and ask it to let you know when it needs more Reiki power to attend to this matter or for other concerns.

Your requests do not have to be limited to spiritual wishes. Also prayers that relate to material goals are completely permissible if they do justice to all the participants. This form of work with your Higher Self is a fantastic opportunity for letting God's will happen here on earth.

Lend a hand and do your part in bringing more love and light to our level. Much of what I have written here probably still appears incomprehensible to you. Don't let yourself be irritated by it and simply start working. Then the lack of insight and misunderstandings will quickly resolve themselves. Both of your "partners" will be glad to help you work with them in the right way. Simply ask them to do so. Everything else then happens practically on its own. Their help is quite likely much more valuable than anything else I could write about the matter.

If you are interested in learning even more about working with the parts of your self, look in the Bibliography. There you will find a number of books on HUNA, which can give you further insights and ideas for your Second Degree work.

Environmental Reiki

The possibilities of Reiki are not at all exhausted with the above applications. With the Second Degree you can also engage in active environmental protection. If you would like to do something about the destruction of the living processes on our planet, you can give Reiki to the entire earth, for example. Or you can concentrate on an area which you know is very damaged. Get together with other Reiki friends who also have the Second Degree and treat a certain area on a regular basis together.

Through the Reiki field created mutually by the group, the energy will flow somewhat more strongly than if each of you were to work alone. In the Appendix, you will find some addresses of organizations in which many Reiki friends have joined together in order to do this important work.

A further useful application for this technique consists of reactivating the earth chakras and earth meridians. Simply establish a connection to the earth chakras and send them Reiki in order to once again normalize their functions. Group work on a regular basis is also the best approach for this purpose.

As a last example, I would like to mention the energetic cleansing of rooms. This application can be arranged in such a way that specific earth rays can be eliminated and others disappear at least for a certain amount of time. Even "technical disturbances,"

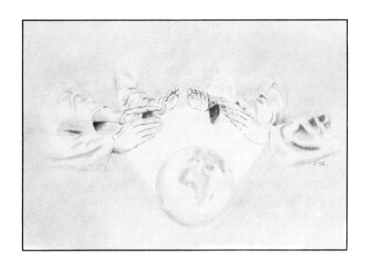

"Environmental Work with Reiki"

if they are not too strong, can be subdued for a time. There is much more that you can do with this tool, but I won't list any further applications at this point. On the one hand, you now have enough ideas to help you develop your own, and on the other hand some of the very intensive applications absolutely require personal instruction and monitoring by an experienced Reiki Master. This work also stands at the center of my Reiki-Do and Rainbow Reiki seminars on the Second Degree, in which more extensive knowledge on these matters is shared.

3. Mental healing

This is one method of having a harmonizing effect on the mental level of a being with the Reiki energy (mental healing).

In this way, a positive influence can be exerted upon fears, disharmonious patterns of behavior, and addictions, among other things.

I still owe you an explanation of the mental level, which I promised you in the above text: You are certainly familiar with the six main chakras of a human being. (If not, they are briefly described in the Appendix). Imagine these energy centers as the horizontal construction of the inner energy structure of a human being. Each of them also has a vertical construction. This can then be subdivided into a number of layers. These levels are given such names as the astral, mental, or ether body. I am only going to deal with the mental body here. It touches all the main chakras and organizes all of the thinking processes, which includes both the conscious and the unconscious. In terms of the main emphasis, important programming occurs during childhood, as well as later, in the mental body. Certain constantly recurrent processes are recognized and retained so that they can automatically be repeated later. This happens when learning to drive a car, for example. At first, you have to think about every shifting process and carry it out quite consciously. Later, everything works automatically. Certain feedback control cycles are assembled, keeping your conscious mind free for current happenings. These automatic behaviors are not only set up for physical procedures, but also for inner ones. For example, this occurs when you have learned from your parents that certain actions, like playing in mud or eating slowly, are undesirable or that work must be strenuous and hostile to pleasure.

Further reflexes, created at a later time, are built on the basis of these restrictions. With time, you have less and less desire to play and eat hastily because you are otherwise confronted with guilt feelings. You are only satisfied with your work if it drains you and you don't have any fun doing it. Even if you perceive at some point that these unconscious thought processes are unhealthy, it will be difficult for you to change them. They are firmly anchored in your subconscious mind (please don't confuse it with your Inner Child!). On the one hand, this arrangement is tremendously practical—there would be no sense in making it easy to change reflexes once they have been learned. On the other hand, because of their enormous perseverance it is very troublesome and tedious to replace the partially decayed substructure of the acquired character qualities through more supportive structures.

Each of us bears a vast quantity of these automatic behaviors within ourselves. We need many of them, but others make our lives more difficult, such as those which time and again have us seek a partner who has looks similar to those of one of our parents because we felt particularly happy with him. This basically is not a problem, but it becomes disruptive when we also treat this partner like our mother or father and have corresponding expectations that are not suitable for a partnership between two adults.

The mental healing technique of the Second Degree is meant to be used for these superfluous, impeding structures that so often grow into quite neurotic vicious circles. In the same simple manner to which you are already accustomed from Reiki, these techniques can help you dissolve such disruptive, subconscious processes and thereby create new freedom for life in the here and now. The conscious, free creation of a life in the present is the indispensable precondition for spiritual growth. Addictions of all types, stagnated concepts of morality, and similar character structures (called "fixations" in psychological terms) that bind you to very specific, harmonious patterns of behavior, thinking, and judging can be simply and harmoniously relaxed and ultimately dissolved.

With this Reiki technique, psychotherapists have a fantastic possibility of helping their patients recover. The fixations are often so dominating that it isn't at all possible to work through the underlying topic. Or an addiction impedes the life situation of the respective person so extremely that he cannot make it through therapy. In these, as well as many other cases based on "false programming" in the subconscious mind, the mental healing method of the Second Degree has proven to be an inestimable help time and again.

However, there are still further useful applications of this technique. You can set up certain automatic behaviors that are holistically sensible (and only these since hypnosis, suggestion, or other "magical" uses are excluded). For this purpose, a good book on affirmations is helpful (my "Chakra Energy Cards," for example—see the Commented Bibliography for further reading recommendations). You can find many ideas there that you can directly apply for your purposes or adapt to your individual needs.

The precondition for fundamental effectiveness is the nonharmful nature of the new automatic behaviors for others and their usefulness for all participants. One example: You want to by a used car and introduce the following thought with the mental healing technique: "I am so eloquent and convincing during a sales conversation that I get the car for a very cheap price." That's not how to do it! Instead, if you use this affirmation: "I permit myself to get a good car that suits my needs at a fair price," the chances for the matter are quite good. With this, you will open yourself up to a fair exchange that is useful to all the participants. To refresh your memory on this topic, you can read back over the section on the "Eternal Laws of Energy Exchange" in the first chapter.

This technique can also be used with an affirmation in order to make very specific things possible or also without one in order to strip away programs that have become superfluous.

One particularly useful method is the selection of affirmations from a pile of cards containing many affirmations for all the important areas of life, according to the principle of chance. You can either make these little cards yourself or use ready-made ones (see lists of sources in the Appendix). Through the "chance" selection, you make it possible for your Higher Self to choose a topic that is particularly important for you at the moment. You can then be certain that you are setting up a new type of program in your subconscious mind that is correct for you in the holistic sense. (It is not helpful to use the pendulum to select such topics! You may want to read the last section about the possibilities of the Inner Child in reference to this.)

This method naturally functions even if you don't use an affirmation. However, with the affirmation cards you have the additional possibility of perceiving the topic important at the moment and then working on it in a carefully directed manner. However, this coincidental method can be associated with one difficulty: perhaps you don't want the answer! Then this technique of mental healing can be restricted in its effectiveness. Similar to the treatment of the body with Reiki, your receptivity also decides on the mental level as to whether Reiki is permitted to flow to you or not.

On the other hand, this situation could be used in a conversational therapy in order to clarify the resistance and its causes. However, another person is required to help you do this. If you would prefer to work on this resistance on your own, think about what you would like to change about your behavior and where it would be easiest for you to do so, meaning where the least amount of resistance can be felt. If you are not familiar with defense mechanisms, read about them in the relevant literature on psychology. Then make yourself a brief, clearly formulated affirmation on your topic and fall back on the suggestions offered by the respective books (see Appendix).

With mental healing, you can also work with the following additional methods: You chose an affirmation card according to the principle of chance after you have prayed for inspiration to help you advance on your path and with which you do not take a defensive attitude when you work with it.

In order to initiate a constant process of learning and transformation for yourself, you can use mental healing without affirmations on a regular basis (at least two to three times per week) for five to ten minutes at a time. This is certainly the path of small steps. Take it and expect nothing so that everything can happen.

All of these possibilities of application should ultimately be organized according to the pleasure principle. Don't create a new straitjacket for yourself, but learn to love yourself by accepting your resistance, learning from it, and then using Reiki in a way that you enjoy. Only then are you taking the Reiki path. Just as you can help yourself with mental healing to break out of the self-imposed vicious circle, you can naturally do the same for others.

Cleansing and charging healing stones with Reiki mental healing

Gemstones can profit from this possibility, as one example. With mental healing you can help them let go of disharmonious programming and accept harmonious programming. This is how they can be cleansed in a far-reaching manner. Even if the conventional cleansing methods like water and sun fail to do the job, the mental technique can reawaken the power of the stone if it has been excessively strained by disharmonious influences, for example.

When you connect this method with the method of distance healing, you can even more intensively help the earth and everything that lives on it at certain points or in general to tune in to the vibration of the New Age and support the concealed potentials that are now so urgently needed.

In summary, it can be said that the mental healing method repeals the limitations of the acquired character structure (active Karma work) and helps you create your conscious and unconscious thought behavior according to the cosmic laws of life.

Personal Growth Through the Second Degree

So—now you know quite well what types of tools the Second Reiki Degree has to offer you. This is necessary in order to understand the opportunities for personal growth that you can put into practice by use of the tools waiting for you.

Important boundaries that many people consider obvious are made relative by the Second Degree.

The energy intensification largely relieves you of the energy flow limitations and thereby brings an enormous reduction in the expenditure of time for the Reiki sessions, which you had to invest during your First Degree phase. The distance treatment techniques will help you overcome the limits of time and space, and the mental healing methods can help you abolish the restrictions set for you by your acquired character structures. Great, isn't it?

And where does it go from here? That's precisely the crux of the matter! You now have a great many tools that cannot be directly abused but only applied for the sake of doing good. It is within your scope of decision-making to use them and set your priorities. You now literally have the possibility in your hands of bring the light and love of God for you and others into this world. Will you do it? How do you feel in the face of this decision? Are you afraid? Are you intoxicated with power? Are you interested in this matter at all, or did you actually prefer to quickly become rich, happy, and famous? You are now in the position of freeing yourself from all the hindering shadows. Your Middle Self can decide on the application of the tools. There are no longer any excuses you can use as a pretext if you remain inactive.

You were powerless, now you no longer are. You were unfree—now you have more possibilities than you ever dreamed of. You have your destiny in your hand and can even help other people on their path. Now you can learn to voluntarily turn to the light, time and again. You do not have to. You can also continue to live like you have up to now and simply act like nothing happened. Or you can decide to grow towards the light and work on yourself. To do this, it is necessary to constantly make yourself aware of why this growth is important.

The beautiful feelings that a Reiki session creates within you are now no longer enough as motivation. Through the possibilities of your mind, you must repeatedly make it clear to yourself why it is important and correct to clarify its structures. Just as the body with its structures was harmonized with the means of the First Degree, the same is now required on the mental and spiritual level. Here, as there, you still have the freedom to say "no" to growth. This is important, since your God-given freedom to make decisions would otherwise be repealed through Reiki. However, Reiki is not meant to take away your freedom, but give you the means to win it for yourself in an extensive manner and use it in the sense of divine consciousness.

Perhaps while reading the section on the applications of the Second Degree tools you already asked yourself where the catch is, where the limitations are: They lie in your will to grow towards God and question yourself frequently in this strenuous process. If you really want to achieve effective results with the mental healing technique, you must learn to continuously see yourself with all your personal value judgments, your moral and ethical concepts, your reflexes in terms of fear, greed, guilt, and morality and question these. In order to continue to grow, it is necessary to dissolve these developed structures.

Love knows no moral restrictions. If your mind wants to learn to love, it must learn to give up its valuations and limitations. The more intensely it risks this, the more it will grow up towards the level of the Higher Self, to contact with God. If it forgets to take its Inner Child along in the process, accept it with its "childish" needs and energies, and learn to love it, it will lose its roots. In this case, the mind cannot apply its potential for the benefit of all beings on this earth since the earthly portions have been excluded from the efforts to grow. Its Inner Child will refuse to give it the energy to live on the earth since it doesn't feel accepted and loved. The Inner Child with its energies like aggression, sexuality, curiosity and joy, play instinct, and the need for closeness cannot be developed away.

With mental healing, you can dissolve the automatic reactions to certain stimuli, but not the source from which these mechanisms receive their energy.

Personal growth with the Second Degree is then a constant balancing act. You have all the possibilities for personal growth, but you can only use them when you apply your will in order to make yourself aware of your limitations. In the process, it is not absolutely necessary to perceive and understand all the disharmonious structures. In the first place, it is necessary to make all your collected theoretical models available through a fundamental decision so that Reiki can develop its healing effect.

As in the First Degree applications, the recipient of the Reiki energy decides whether and to what extent he will "absorb" it.

If you are basically not willing to let go of your moral concepts and patterns of behavior, Reiki will not take away your freedom to continue to live with them. But if you are inwardly willing to also let your mental level be penetrated by the divine, loving light, Reiki will effectively help you in doing so.

Ultimately, it is a conscious decision and, similar to the First Degree, you can do certain exercises in the Second Degree in order to make it easier for you to let go of your claims to power.

But even here, you are not yet finished. The mental healing technique will help you dissolve disharmonious structures. Afterwards, you must establish new, more harmonious ones since you cannot live without structures. You have been incarnated on the level of a variety of structures. But where should you get them? An important orientation guide for you could be the five Reiki life principles, as well as the ancient books of wisdom like the Chinese I Ching oracle with its timeless messages about the nature of the world.

In case of doubt, you can always ask your Higher Self for advice when you establish a Reiki connection with it.

It was important for me personally to explore the history of humanity and the many different civilizations that it has produced. The more you become familiar with all the variations of moral and ethical structures, the more difficult it will be for you to judge your current opinion to be the only reasonable one.

Millions of people have thought and acted in a way different from yours, and they also achieved a great deal for themselves and their fellow human beings. Two examples should give you thought-provoking impulses for your own involvement with this topic: In certain North American Indian tribes, it was a part of becoming an adult that adolescents left the protective community of the tribe for a while and searched for their power animal and their spiritual vision. Completely alone, they sometimes spent many weeks in the wilderness, were hungry and at the mercy of the weather and the wild animals. Many died in this search. This type of self-discovery was considered absolutely necessary on the path to becoming an adult human being.

If something like this would happen today, the society as a whole would attack the cruel people who subjected their poor, helpless children to such needless suffering and dangers.

Some peoples who were still in harmony with nature had the same expression for "having sex with each other" and "becoming acquainted with someone." In daily life, this meant a much less constrained approach to sexual contacts than what we are accustomed to today. At the same time, these people had no words for "war" or "crime." Since these types of behavior did not exist, there also were no terms to describe them...

Exercises for Personal Growth with the Methods of the Second Degree

Reiki treatments on a regular basis are an important exercise for you. They ensure that physical tensions are quickly reduced before they become established and can impede you in your mental and spiritual growth. However, they are also there so that the physical blocks that have been created through the Reiki work on the related mental structures can be dissolved and not have the indirect effect of re-establishing certain disharmonious reflexes.

The Second Degree techniques permit you to enormously shorten your sessions so that you increase your free time, which you can use in part to work on mental structures (mental treatment) or work through your past in this and other lives. This is also an opportunity to establish contacts with your Higher Self or your Inner Child (distance treatment).

For me, Reiki treatments are practiced on a regular basis: at least three times a week for 20 minutes. Even better are 30 minutes a day, particularly if you are starting with the personality work of the Second Degree. An hour once a month is not worth it! It is also a wonderful experience to give yourself a 90-minute distance treatment with much energy intensification at some point. It can be like an energy bath and will probably be among the most beautiful and moving experiences of your life.

A further exercise is oracle work with Tarot, runes, or the I Ching. With the help of your Higher Self, which directs these oracles, find out which of the acquired character structures most severely obstructs your development at the moment and then work on dissolving it with the mental healing technique.

In this work, a good aid can be the affirmation cards and books mentioned above. You can also have significant experiences with the "what if...?" exercise.

Take a good hour of your time and write down what consequences there would be for your life if you could turn certain moral concepts or other fixations that you particularly cling to into their exact opposite.

If you cannot imagine how you could live in such a way, look in books, films, or magazines for descriptions of people who do just that. They always exist, you can be sure of it!

Contacts with your Inner Child and your Higher Self on a regular basis can help you understand your personality with all its facets and possibilities as a whole and learn to love it.

The contacts do not need to take place more often than once a week for five to ten minutes respectively, except if you desire to establish the connections to your partners more frequently.

Last but not least, turn to the chapter on the First Degree and read the section on the Reiki life principles time and again, as well as the related practical exercises. Collect experiences with them and get accustomed to practicing on a regular basis.

Summary

Even more than in the First Degree, you assume responsibility for your own life with the conscious use of the Second Degree for the promotion of your personal growth. You can cause yourself to no longer be just a plaything of the external powers of the present and of the burden from your past life, but the master of your destiny within the scope of the universal context, of which your path in life is an important component.

The more you work with the possibilities of the Second Degree, the more applications you will discover and the more familiar you will become with the new, more extensive view of the world that you will get to know in this manner. In the process, do not expect your life to change radically from one day to the next. Although this may happen, it is quite rare. If you apply Reiki according to the pleasure principle, which means always giving Reiki when you feel like it and not when you don't feel like it, you will become involved in a growth process that completely suits you in both its tempo and its manner. If your changes are to take place harmoniously, your body must also have the time to adapt itself since it sometimes is much slower than your mind.

Your partner, your friends and acquaintances, your relatives, and colleagues all will need time to get used to the new person and learn to cope with you. If you radically confront them with new opinions and ways of living according to the motto: "Why should I care about these backwards people?," their reaction will not be particularly friendly and they will put obstacles in your path in one way or another. Perhaps they simply will no longer want to have anything to do with you.

If you get into such a situation, you will notice because of what the others reflect back to you that you have taken on too much. Through their behavior, they show you important parts of your personality that are not yet able to cope with the new attitudes.

Let yourself grow harmoniously according to your own tempo. This type of development is much more sound and extensive than the "Illumination in 30 Days" method.

It could very much be that you still must and want to go through many experiences from the realm of the First Degree, even after you have already received the Second Degree. This is completely correct and normal. The Reiki path is not organized in terms of a hierarchy, but holographically. In principle, all aspects exist in each of the degrees, although they may have different points of emphasis and present them from a different perspective. But you have the freedom to gather your experiences where you like.

It is not necessary to first work through all the areas of the First Degree in order to become initiated into the Second Degree! This is no more necessary than having all the experiences in the area of "personality development" made possible by the Second Degree before you are initiated into the Third Degree. Although there are certain preconditions for the Third Degree, and they are generally examined in a certain respect in contrast to the first two degrees before you are initiated to become a Master, the developmental possibilities depicted in the two last chapters present only a portion of this.

You can also have things to learn in the area of "accepting feelings" or "letting go of claims to power" as a Reiki Master and still be a "good" Master. This topic will be elaborated on in the next chapter about the development of the personality, which can be sparked by the Third Degree.

Instructional Sentences for the Second Degree

Time and again, you should become aware of the consequences which result in relation to your image of the world because the existence of the Second Degree abilities. Learn to see your value judgments and other concepts of how the world should be in a relative sense.

Replace the terms "good" and "bad" with "meaningful for me at this time!" and "I can't perceive the meaning for me at the moment!" when you talk or think about something.

Any affirmations that you give yourself in order to attain more harmonious mental structures are never perfect, but in any case more meaningful for you at the time than the previous ones.

Take the contact to your Higher Self and your Inner Child seriously. The first can be the best teacher you have ever had, and the other the best playmate and friend.

Time and again, you should become aware that power without love, as well as love without power, means death.

With all of your abilities, there is ultimately only one person you can change—yourself!

As long as you want to change the outer world without changing your inner world at least as intensively, you obstruct every type of true growth towards the light.

You are good and correct, lovable and healthy. You just have to allow yourself to be it!

No one is wiser than you if you accept your own wisdom!

Chapter Five

Third Degree Reiki

Why Does Someone Want to Become a Reiki Master?

There are a great variety of expectations. One of them is to become more holy, which is nonsense. Even after a Master initiation, a person with strengths and weaknesses is still a person with strengths and weaknesses.

Another expectation is one of receiving the ultimate wisdom, which is just as incorrect. Each person must still search for and discover this alone.

Other people think it would be a great job to just work on a few weekends and earn a pile of money in the process. In addition, they could become famous, respected, and finally be loved. Here as well, this expectation cannot necessarily be realized. If a person had problems before with money, love, and a feeling of self-worth, he will continue to have them as a Reiki Master. The only difference is that he will have to confront these difficulties even more frequently and more intensively.

One last expectation is that of learning something more about oneself and also using these experiences to help others discover and learn to love themselves. An entire spectrum of mixtures of these expectations exist—just as many as there are people. Very rarely will you meet someone who has a pure form of one of these attitudes of expectancy.

Thank God, the high price stops most people with rather superficial ideas about the life of a Reiki Master from risking the step and venturing the training. At the same time, this is also an explanation on the amount of return service for the Master initiation. Hawayo Takata took $10,000. for it. This was a gigantic sum of money in those days, something like the annual wage of a middle-level employee. Takata-Sensei once said that someone who wants to become a Reiki Master must be willing to give up everything he owns. I believe she did not mean that this person

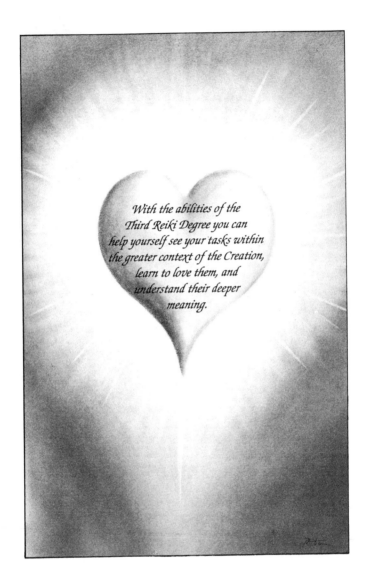

With the abilities of the Third Reiki Degree you can help yourself see your tasks within the greater context of the Creation, learn to love them, and understand their deeper meaning.

should give everything to her if he wants to become a Master, but rather that he should examine his willingness to make available all possessions, all obligations, and everything he believes he knows about the world. He should be willing to let it all go.

A hand that holds onto something cannot grasp something new, a glass that is already full cannot receive any new liquid—these are wise old sayings. For a person who would like to become a Reiki Master, they have great meaning. Personal development during the Third Degree in particular succeeds or fails with the willingness to learn how to let go. Only then will it be possible for God—or however you want to call THIS DIVINE FORCE—to help and guide your Higher Self.

Perhaps you are now asking yourself why this matter is so important to me. In my time as a Master, I have learned that this occupation (calling) is not particularly easy, that it makes invaluable experiences possible for myself and others, and that it is very important to stay standing with both feet on the ground of reality when the job consists of passing on the energy of Heaven. The more illusions and expectations you have about the effects of the Master initiation, the more difficult it will be for you to cope with the new reality when you are a Master.

The less secure your stance is, the more easily you will start to waver in the face of racing developments. But before we go into more detail on this topic, I would like to describe the course of the Reiki Master training to you.

What Happens in a Traditional Master Training?

Once you have had experiences with the Second Degree over a longer period of time of at least one year (in my opinion) and have learned to use the tools with great certainty, then you can approach a Master whom you trust and ask to be trained for the Third Degree.

You can naturally already try to find someone who will take you into the training beforehand, but you should give some exact thought to whether you are cheating yourself in this case. For every degree, you should necessarily take a certain amount of time to collect experiences with its possibilities in order to fundamentally learn to deal with the new abilities and your reactions to the energies released in the Reiki work.

It is by no means enough to just become familiar with what your mind can comprehend about Reiki. Very much—I think almost everything—takes place at the intuitive level, in the realm of the emotions when you deal with the universal life energy. Developments there need much longer than the experiences that the mind can comprehend in order to be worked through and truly become a new component of the personality.

For the First Degree, you need at least two to three months. For the Second Degree, at least a year is required in order to integrate the experiences with the respective form of Reiki work. The precondition is that you occupy yourself with the energy on a regular basis and in a conscious manner.

But let's assume that you become a Master within a shorter amount of time. Other people will then come to you so that you can initiate them and explain to them how they can use the universal life energy. They will have many questions for you that can only be answered on the basis of practical experience and not by rote from books you have read.

It will also be a part of your duties to explain how to use the symbols and mantras of the Second Degree. What are you going to do if you cannot yet deal with these things yourself and cannot answer questions because you don't have the practical experience and possibly even the necessary knowledge? You may be able to fool the Master who trains you to a certain degree, but not your students!

Let's assume you have adequately confronted the possibilities of the first two degrees and had a certain amount of experience with them. What now? First, think about which Master you would like to go to. This question is enormously important. You should have a good feeling about him. This is the foundation for your trust. Without a solid relationship of trust between you, the Master cannot train you.

During the training to become a Reiki Master, situations of open or concealed tensions will occur between the two of you time and again. This is a part of the training. If the emotional bond between the two of you is not strong enough, in the case of an intense strain you will either discontinue the training with this Master and thereby deprive yourself of a very important learning experience or you will put on an act and try to hide your true feelings according to the motto: "In a few months I'll be a Master myself and then he can go to hell...!"

The training becomes a farce with this mental attitude. Perhaps you will succeed in deceiving the Master if you are a good actor and he is not particularly attentive for some reason, but you will also be deceiving yourself.

The Development of the Personality in the Master Training

The initiation to be a Master cannot and should not relieve you of any personal learning experiences! If you do not know the Master you want to train you, it is recommended that you get to know him personally before you make your final decision. You should also visit one or two of his seminars as a guest. If you feel a strong inner connection to the Master, he is probably the right one for you.

In this process, it is not necessary to think everything he does is wonderful. It is more important for you to be able to accept him as a person, even if you notice any rough edges he may have. If you have found the right Master for you and have been accepted by him as a student, you will be present at many of his seminars as a guest or even as an assistant in order to enter into the Master energy more intensely.

Through the experiences with continuously new Reiki groups and changed basic conditions, you can learn what it actually takes to have a good Reiki seminar. With time, you will better perceive the manner in which your Reiki Master holds seminars and treats the students. This will help you become clear about what you would like to assume from him and what you would like to do differently. In this way, you will find your own vision of Reiki with time.

This vision cannot be found without the long training relationship with your Master. It is therefore not particularly helpful if you already have fixed ideas about it in advance and then take the training. Only the personal contact with your trainer can truly permit this—*your*—vision of the path as a Reiki Master to develop.

During the training period, you should also clarify your relationship to very fundamental things like money, love, relationships, closeness, power, envy, greed, and so forth. In this process, it is certainly not necessary to completely cope with everything. It is much more your task to learn to know yourself, perceive what you can deal with and what causes you difficulties.

Perfection is not a precondition for the Third Reiki Degree. If it were, there would be no Reiki Masters. But you should be as honest as possible with yourself. This sincerity can be an invaluable help to you later when you are a Master.

No one is more securely under God's protection than someone who can disclose his own mistakes and own up to them when this is necessary.

At some point during your time as an apprentice, you will quite automatically project your father or mother relationship onto your master. This is also important, and this is precisely the point when proof will be given of whether the trust between the two of you is strong enough to make the pending learning process possible. If you oriented yourself on your parents as a child and accepted everything they told you was good and right, there will also be a time when you shape the relationship to your Master to fit in with this concept. After a certain amount of time, you will fall into the other extreme. Suddenly, everything he does is nonsense. "How can a person be like that!" you will probably think.

Now you are in the phase of defiance. This is also a completely normal and important development. It is important to have free space and create the possibility for yourself of defining the limits between yourself and your trainer, finding your own "self" as a Reiki Master. This is the time in which students most often discontinue the training. It is quite possible that some ugly scenes happen between the two of you, but your trainer will repeatedly open the door for you when you want to go to him, and otherwise let you go your own way. Perhaps you openly or secretly accuse him of being an impossible person who has not yet initiated you because of a lack of insight or out of pure malice, although you have long been mature enough to become a Reiki Master, maybe even more mature than he.

After some time, which could be weeks or months, you will see more clearly. You will perceive that every person is different and has a good right to be different. You will be able to permit your Master to be himself and thereby show that you have accepted yourself in an important point: you can now believe in yourself and your own path! This development is the foundation for the energy of the initiation, which will be at hand in the near future. When both of you, you and your Master, agree that the time is ripe for your initiation into the Third Degree, you will mutually establish a time period of three or four days during which the great event should occur.

However, before this happens at least one year can and should pass. Perhaps there are only the two of you, or perhaps there are also further Third Degree students present when you come together for the Master seminar. It can be that a self-discovery seminar may take place some days beforehand, in which clarification can be achieved. Sometimes one person or the other will notice at the last moment that it still isn't the right time for him and leaves before the actual Master course. Those who feel themselves ready, and are also evaluated as such by the trainers, will then meet together and usually receive the initiation into the Third Degree and the Master symbol right at the start.

There will then be several days of intensive learning. It is quite important to know by heart the rituals of the initiation into the Reiki degrees and also securely master all the mantras and symbols. During these classes, the courses of the first two degrees are often discussed as well in order to eliminate any possible unclear points and to prepare the new Masters as well as possible for their work. Each graduate of this course receives a certificate from the training Master so the student can prove that he has been initiated accordingly into the Third Degree of the Usui System of Reiki in the traditional manner and trained for the work of a Master.

The Approach to the Universal Life Energy and the Tradition of the Usui System of Natural Healing

A further important partial area of training in the Master/Teacher Degree is the personal approach of the student to Reiki and to the tradition of the method. For this purpose, it is necessary to deal with the great variety of Reiki application possibilities in both theory and practice. It is important to come into contact with the universal life force time and again under the direction of an experienced trainer: to experience its short-term and long-term effects on health, the body, the psyche, and spiritual development on oneself and others and to analyze and learn to accept it on a gut level. It is also just as important to understand and learn to use the special laws that characterize the Reiki energy work. Reiki is a very special power and its effects cannot simply just be equated with those of polarity, shiatsu, prana healing, or forms of faith healing.

A future Reiki Master must absolutely know what Reiki *cannot* do and where the limitations of this method lie so that he can correctly and realistically advise students and clients. An extensive general knowledge of anatomy, physiology, pathology, psychology, psychotherapy, group dynamics, essential esoteric theoretical models, and the laws of holistic healing, as well as knowledge of relevant legal regulations on questions of healing are also desirable. The second Grand Master of Reiki, the physician Dr. Chujiro Hayashi, took these last two points particularly seriously and give his students extensive instruction on them. For example, he sent Hawayo Takata, whom he later named to be his successor, to a famous Japanese health resort for a number of months so that she could supplement her studies at his clinic and further expand her knowledge about methods of natural healing.

In my opinion, it is only possible to walk the Reiki path— particularly as a Master—by repeatedly becoming involved with the history of the Usui System of Natural Healing and understanding and practicing Dr. Usui's path, including the problems and the solutions he found for them. Dr. Usui's search for a spiritual method of healing, the way in which he found this unbelievably valuable treasure, and the form that he developed after a number of failed attempts in order to correctly treat the process of healing and impart the system to others, has been and continues to be an inexhaustible source of vitally important impulses and perceptions for my own private and professional path. According to my experience, Dr. Usui's principles of healing and life and his way of teaching Reiki are just as valid today as they were back then. This also applies to studying the symbols and mantras of the Usui System, and the emotional, mental, and spiritual approach to these essential tools.

126

The Harmonization of Personal Problem Fields in the Scope of the Master Training

I find that the third and last essential aspect of the Master training is a re-orientation of the student's way of life. It is not necessary—and not even possible—to "cure" all the problems within this period of time. But a change should occur within the Master student in the direction of considerably greater flexibility, clearly more liveliness, and the enthusiasm for continuous learning in all areas. A Reiki Master should not have "already learned everything," but be willing to learn to discover the world anew each day and give up yesterday's convictions that no longer function in accordance with life in favor of more suitable mental attitudes. Then—and only then—can Reiki increasingly flow within and through the student, enriching his private life and work.

I have developed the principles described here on the basis of practical experience. For more than five years (as of 1996), I have trained Reiki Masters in one-to-two-year training periods with more than 600 hours of instruction at my Reiki-Do Institute. There has been—and still is—much for me to learn in this process, and time and again I have the opportunity of immediately examining innovations in terms of their suitability in the practice. As a result, one question has proved to be very important: "If I were a Master student right here and now in this program, would I really be able to learn everything in terms of personal and professional contents that I will absolutely need afterwards in my professional practice as a Reiki Master in order to be a good teacher to my students and be happy with my own path?" Try to use this question as orientation for yourself on your path to becoming a Reiki Master in order to test the suitability of training programs and—later—in the training of your own students. You will quickly discover: it's a question worth asking for the benefit of all participants involved.

At the end of this section, I would like to address a question that is frequently posed by Master students with "previous training." It's something like this:

"I'm a doctor and psychotherapist who has worked with holistic methods for years and I have also been thoroughly involved with esoterics for years. I personally participated in psychotherapy for more than four years. And in addition to this, I've completed nine different types of therapeutic training. Why should I actually spend another 12 or more months on a Reiki Master training program? I can already do everything. Can't you just initiate me right away?"

My answer to this is:

"It's wonderful that you've made so much of your life up to now. You've really made an effort to take this aphorism to heart: The path is the goal! I think it would be great if you continue being true to your motto. Use the 12 or more months of the Master training to apply everything you are and can do for the exploration of the Reiki path. Because you don't know *it* yet. Even if you have travelled in a hundred countries, a new, unknown country will only reveal its special characteristics and beauty to you if you take the time to explore it. Enjoy its air, taste its water, cross it on foot, live with its inhabitants, and get to know their manners and customs.

Flying over it, taking pictures, pasting the airline ticket into the album, and then boasting to friends about a further land that you're "acquainted with" is tourism in fits and starts."

Opportunities for Growth with the Third Degree Reiki

You will probably first notice after the Master seminar that the increase in energy was much stronger than in your wildest dreams. You will probably be so full of energy that you have the feeling of constantly lifting off. For this reason, it is recommended that you take some vacation time after the Third Degree course. Pay a great deal of attention to yourself and get used to the new qualities of your personal energy. You will notice that everything is somehow different. You have been given fantastic abilities and can create a solid connection to God's healing powers for anyone who would like them.

Yet, you are still the person you were before. There's no halo shining over your head, your finger will still bleed if you cut it while making a salad, and you still will not be able to pull the answers to all the important and inconsequential questions of your life out of the hat. You will spend the rest of your life with this (apparent) paradox. Grant yourself the time to get used to it before you give courses and have to confront new situations.

As a Reiki Master, you essentially "just" have one more ability in your tool kit than someone with the Second Degree: you can impart to other people a lasting connection to the source of universal life energy and transmit to them a great variety of ways of dealing with it. This makes quite clear what prospects the Third Degree offers for personal development: you must initiate other people and show them what they can do with the Reiki power! You will grow and continue to develop as a result of this process.

Because of these circumstances, I don't think much of initiating people into the Third Degree without transmitting to them the knowledge for all the initiations and the Master symbol. Although it is claimed that this 3A level is meant for people who only want to use the Master energy for their own personal development, precisely this is not what is promoted here, with the exception of the strong "energy kick" of the Third Degree initiation. This means that the activity for which the Master Degree was conceived cannot even be pursued. However, like everything else in this book, this is my personal viewpoint and does not necessarily apply to you. Come up with your own ideas about it and find your own standpoint. This is more important than assuming my opinion.

The Seminars

As a Master, you will experience the courses of the First and Second Degrees from a completely different perspective. You are suddenly the person who is being asked the questions, who ultimately supports and shapes the seminar. On the basis of your example, the students will orient themselves in relation to how they deal with Reiki and many other aspects of their lives as well. In every seminar, you will feel the presence and the help of God and the ascended Grand Masters of Reiki. You will channel the enormous energy necessary to transform a person into a Reiki channel. The constant intensive contact with the heavenly power will change your life at least as intensively as the unique experience of the Master initiation. After each seminar, you will float on the clouds or even be quite down because there were many unpleasant things for you to learn.

Perhaps you will gain a few kilos of weight during the next months because these pounds are necessary to "ground" you until you have found another possibility for this purpose. It is naturally also possible that either no participants or very few come to your courses. What will you do then? Did you already plan on the money because you took out a loan for the Master initiation? Have you possibly already quit your job because you think you no longer need a "normal" occupation? This is how your Higher Self can show you that your idea of relationships, material things like money or other fundamental structures need further clarification.

Go to work on it and find a good therapist (in case you don't have one) in order to discover new paths for yourself. Work with the methods of the First and Second Degrees in order to support the necessary growth processes. This is an excellent opportunity for coming to yourself. Don't put the blame on others. Stay with yourself, and you will notice that there are suddenly paths where only impenetrable jungles were before. Then your courses will also have a better rate of attendance. If you can inwardly stand up for what you show to the outside, others can also trust in you and turn to you.

This developmental step also belongs to the Third Degree. Not everyone experiences this so dramatically, but at some point each individual must find out what his path is. The orientation for this purpose should be planned during the Third Degree training. The fine tuning on one's own path after the Master initiation then lasts for the rest of your life. Through the constant intensive contact with Reiki, each Master will be stimulated into liveliness time and again. The more you defend yourself against this development, the more difficult it will be for you. The more intensively you let go of your personal claims to power, the more beautiful and harmonious the developments in your life will be.

Your first learning situations when your courses are full will also be involved with these claims to power and love, closeness, and money. When I began my activities as a Reiki Master and immediately had plenty of students, I was involved in two car accidents within 10 days. And this happened to me despite the fact that I had driven up to 100,000 kilometers a year without any accidents! Both times I slid for some inexplicable reason into another car at a snail's pace. Since the insurance required a high percentage excess in both cases, I had to pay a lot of money—just about what I had earned through the previous seminars. Later, I then understand the cause of these annoying incidents: Although I could manage well with the relationship to the students, I could not yet permit myself to accept the energy exchange, the money, for my services.

Your Students—Your Mirror

All the people who come to you in order to be initiated into a Reiki degree have a message for you. This is not what they say, but a characteristic trait, a quality, or a question they pose for you.

During the Reiki seminar, each of your students reflects a part of your personality that you have not yet truly learned to accept and love. The more attentively you treat your students, the more you take them seriously, the more likely it is that this message will be revealed to you. Phyllis Lei Furumoto, the current Grand Master of the Reiki Alliance, has coined this phrase: "I thank you for being my teacher!". This sentence relates to her students. Try to live the relationship to your students with a similar attitude, and they will be fantastic and loving teachers for you.

One topic that I would still like to illuminate is how to deal with power. Every Reiki Master has a great deal of it. By power, I don't mean the power to initiate other people to be Reiki channels. You have only borrowed this power—it is fundamentally performed by God. No, I'm talking about the power to be the top dog, shining example, guru, or something similar for other people who would like to have this and confuse the function of "Reiki Master" (which is divine and perfect) with the personality that is human and just as imperfect as that of any other human being.

The temptation to fall for this game is great, and it's probably a part of life to try it for a while. But the reality will bring you back down to earth (and humanity) sooner or later (usually sooner).

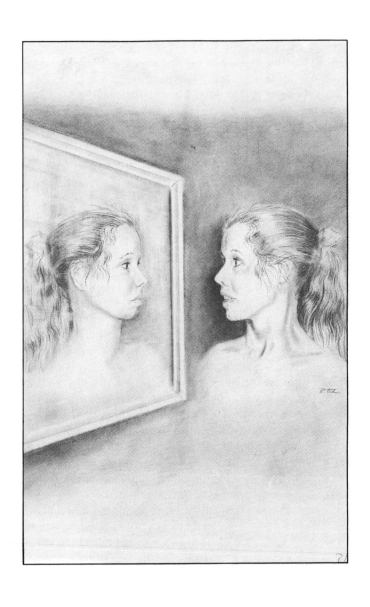

*As a Reiki Master, you will be confronted with your mirror image
time and again ...*

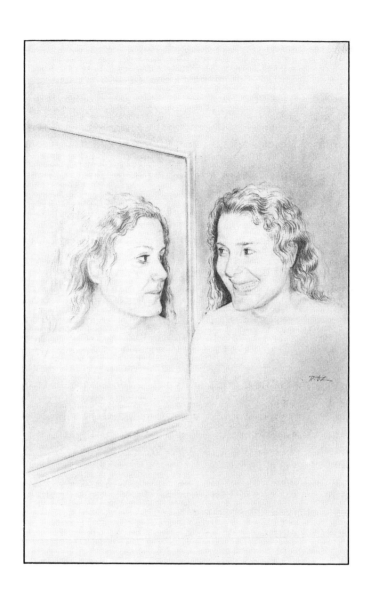

... and this is how you can learn to love yourself and become whole.

However, the landing can be much softer if you have become sensitive to this problem in time. I solve this power situation by questioning my infallibility right at the start of every seminar, as obviously as possible and at all possible opportunities. In addition, despite all my personal efforts on behalf of my standpoint, I declare my viewpoints to be personal valuations and not eternal wisdom. And yet, I still fall into the trap time and again if someone is skillful enough in offering me the opportunity. But the landing is softer, and I can also laugh about my "unteachableness" in the meantime.

The more you "walk in the clouds," the more you will distance yourself from human closeness, warm-hearted relationships to other people, the small and yet so important and irreplaceable joys of everyday life. At the beginning, you can quite consciously permit yourself a few flights of fancy so that you can grasp as quickly as possible: "Down with the others it's much more pleasant in the long run." The best helpers on your path as a Master can be your students, your friends, and your acquaintances. Particularly the friends who have nothing to do with esoterics, and for this reason do not look at you with eyes transfigured by the initiation, can be quite helpful. Or those who have their initiation behind them for some time already and have thereby gained more distance to you. With distance, I don't mean less love (which usually grows with time), but distance to assuming your perspective of the world without a comment.

I hope these short scenes from my growth experiences will help you on your path.

In the meantime, I believe the essential things that a person must learn are the same for everyone. Each of us just seeks different paths and times to become familiar with them.

Reiki Work for Yourself

I first had to learn to get used to the work on the weekends and evenings, taking and permitting myself leisure time on other occasions. This time for yourself is particularly important after a seminar. You will need some space to digest the experiences and become conscious of all the important things that happened for you during the course. Letting go of the claims and questions by the students is also important. Now you are once again yourself and you should live your own life. In these free hours, you should also take time for a continuation of the Reiki work on yourself. It is particularly important in the Third Degree to be intensively involved with Reiki outside of the courses and establish an exchange with your Inner Child and/or Higher Self using the techniques of the Second Degree. The intensification of your own sensitivity and new experiences time and again through the contact with Reiki can be an inestimable gain for not only yourself, but for your students as well. The more you are capable of perceiving energies and differentiating their qualities, the better you can address the questions that are behind the questions your students ask. This will help you better perceive the mirror image that they have in store for you.

One last word about the so-called "Master energy." In all degrees of the Reiki method, work is done exclusively with *one* quality of life energy—Reiki. This is where the system gets its name. In the First Degree, the way of fundamentally opening up to and applying this power is imparted. In the Second Degree, three special tools are transmitted: one for the intensification and spatial orientation of Reiki, another for the direct transmission of Reiki on the mental level of the human energy body, and another for the transmission of Reiki to other living beings independent of time and space. One further symbol and a mantra is added in the Third Degree.

Both of these instruments are necessary in order to carry out the initiations in all three degrees. This means that for the Reiki Masters there is no special healing power that goes beyond the abilities of the students in the First or Second Degrees. More frequently it is probably the higher degree of experience in using Reiki and holistic healing, as well as strong charisma created by the intensive work on one's own personality and the activity of a leadership position, which can naturally have a positive influence on the client's receptivity for Reiki. Yet, I have often enough experienced people who had "just" been initiated into the First Degree but had completely extraordinary healing success with Reiki and possessed a very strong, loving personality.

If you are interested in doing the Master training because you believe the healing business only really starts at that point, you are totally mistaken! In this case, the best advice is for you to visit advanced training for the First and Second Degrees, collect a great deal of practical experience with Reiki, explore the laws of holistic healing, and learn to understand the principles according to which this wonderful power functions.

When I write about the "Master energy" in this book, what I mean is the sometimes quite hefty effects of the initiation into the Third Degree on the one hand and the special art of personality development experienced by a Reiki Master who devotes himself to this calling, as well as the personal power and charisma which result.

The purpose of this chapter should be to create more understanding for the path of the Reiki Master on the part of people who are initiated into the First or Second Degree and to help avoid false expectations. If you are not yet a Master, but are playing with the thought of taking this beautiful path, this chapter can then offer you an initial orientation. Like everything else in this book, this portrayal of the training and path of a Reiki Master also represents what I know and think about the topic. You should in any case talk about the Third Degree with one or more Reiki Masters if you are considering taking this path.

I look forward to a future when there is a competent Reiki Master in every town. This lovely way of accessing the universal life energy will then be a part of our everyday lives and be more easily available for many people.

Perhaps you would also like to join in the work of putting the energy of heaven into the hands of the people on earth. Then don't hesitate to take this path.

Summary

The purpose of the Third Degree is to clarify and develop your spiritual self, which in plain English means: learning to understand, experience, and accept your place in the creation, your relationship to God and the power of God's love.

Additional Remarks

The question arises frequently for many people as to whether Reiki Masters shouldn't have a license as a non-medical practitioner or a physician's degree since they do teach other people to heal. From my perspective, this is not absolutely necessary. It is certainly useful for a Reiki Master to have fundamental knowledge of anatomy, physiology, and pathology. But more than sound general knowledge is not required.

In the strict sense, Reiki is less a method of healing in medical terms than a method of developing the personality on all levels. One of the "side effects" is that physical symptoms are resolved when the respective people grow out of the psychological structures that are their underlying basis. If participants have questions on specific medical problems during the seminars, it is not necessary and (in most countries) not even legally permissible to answer them.

In the first place, people who are neither naturopaths nor doctors are not permitted to give diagnoses or prescribe therapies; in the second place, it would not be very responsible to distribute advice from the palm of your hand. In such a case, it would be better to pass on the address of a good specialist who can and is permitted to attend to specific medical problems. A Reiki seminar is meant to essentially impart knowledge about the transmission of universal life energy that is applicable without any major problems for each individual; it is not meant to replace a private consultation session. A well-trained Reiki Master is always qualified for the first situation. He may also be qualified for the other situation, but doesn't have to be.

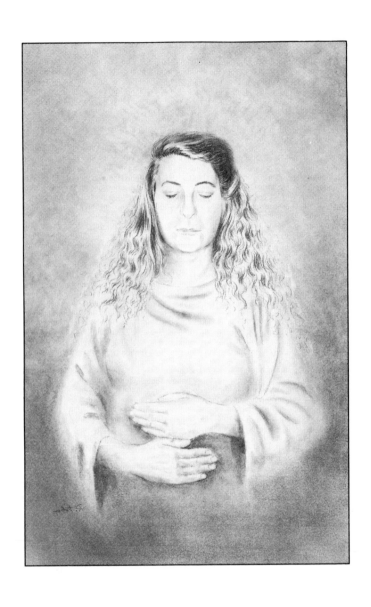

Reiki should initially be there for you once you have become a Reiki channel. Only when you have time to spare should you treat friends and relatives.

Chapter Six

What About Further Degrees?

The System of the T.R.T.A.I.

As mentioned at the end of the last chapter, there are also other ways of looking at the path of a Reiki Master. I would like to introduce some of them here as representative of the many others which are similar in nature. One of these is represented by the T.R.T.A.I., the Reiki organization headed by the Grand Master Dr. Barbara Weber (see Chapter One, section on "The History of the Usui System of Reiki"). Since the T.R.T.A.I. has had the greatest influence on the modern history of Reiki, in addition to the Reiki Alliance, here is a brief introduction to its approach. This organization has an established training plan for Master candidates. Since about 1985, it has initiated people into four further degrees, making a total of seven. At this point in time, Dr. Weber announced that she had been the only one to receive further symbols, mantras, and the methods for applying these from Takata-Sensei. There are greatly differing rumors about these symbols in addition to the official version.

After a number of years of intensive research on my part and the further theoretic and practical study of the Usui System of Natural Healing, I have come to the conclusion that additional degrees and everything related to them are probably Dr. Weber's own development. In any case, there are no serious indications of further degrees before she began propagating them. Furthermore, the system of the three degrees is completely perfect within itself.

On the one hand, the meaning of the Master symbols is a symbolic repetition of Dr. Usui's initiation experience on the holy mountain Kurgyama; on the other hand, they are a description of the Buddha nature. In the ritual of the Master initiation, the Buddha nature and the Buddha consciousness are made applicable for the initiated Reiki Master in relation to their transmission for the awakening of the connected healing power. This is the greatest gift that can be made accessible to a human being—without personal efforts! Even outside the channeled transmission of the healing powers, a personal development into a Buddha nature (which means the practical realization of the Buddha nature and consciousness in everyday life) can only be achieved through personal exertion and lengthy learning processes. An initiation can *in no way* have this effect. Human beings are ultimately not machines.

At the same time, it is not my opinion that no additional symbols and mantras should be included in the classic Reiki system. I therefore do not doubt the effectiveness of the further initiations of the T.R.T.A.I. But I also have no indication that these or similar expansions of the Usui System of Natural Healing are principally something other than additional subdivisions of the Second Degree. This means there is nothing that cannot also be done with the three classical symbols and their mantras when used in a competent manner. There are no additional energies in the Usui System of Natural Healing—the type of effects can be clearly defined and set apart from other forms of energy work.

In addition, Dr. Usui said that he heals with Reiki and not with X-ki, Y-ki, or Z-ki as well. In this respect, further initiations, mantras, and symbols can either help to purposefully send Reiki into various areas of the subtle energy system or other levels of existence, as in the example of what happens through the distance healing symbol and the mental healing symbol—or they belong to another system of energy work in which powers other than Reiki are employed. The latter case can be very appropriate, but to call this Reiki only confuses and complicates effective and systematic energy work. Like every other form of life energy, Reiki also has very definite principles according to which it behaves. This topic will be discussed in detail later in the chapter.

By the way, I am open at any time to information that suggests other conclusions in a verifiable manner. I enjoy learning.

Since the T.R.T.A.I. introduced further degrees, much water—and other things—has flowed down the Missouri River and a series of other Reiki Masters came up with similar ideas, introducing further symbols and degrees. What should we make of these particular cases? After I carefully examined the tradition to see if this type of thing could be found anywhere—and discovered nothing—I experimented with the Reiki techniques of the Second and

Third Degrees in order to introduce additional symbols and mantras I had selected to the Usui System of Natural Healing in addition to the traditional ones.

It took a while, but then I got the hang of it and could initiate some volunteers into symbols and mantras which directed Reiki right into the various chakras or the aura fields, karmic areas, the angel levels, the shamanic lower and upper worlds, or the elementary energy fields. I was quite euphoric for a while, but after I had thoroughly thought things through and tried them out, I decided not to publish the results of my research work or pass them on to my students. Why not? It's quite simple: Everything that you could engage in with the additional tools (mantras and symbols) can be done just as well with the traditional three instruments of the Second Degree.*

The more symbols and mantras we use, the more complicated the ingeniously simple and unbelievably flexible Usui System of Reiki becomes, in my opinion. In addition, the students of this method quickly dissipate their energies in a forest of symbols and have less opportunities to grasp the vast spiritual depth and the enormous possibilities of the three tools of the Second Degree. There is already enough confusion in this respect.

One further point that caused me to make my decision is something that I call the "initiation mentality." People who have this mental attitude collect initiations, symbols, mantras, and other "holy stuff" in the belief that this will help them get a grip on their life without any greater efforts on their part. They think that through this form of hoarding behavior alone they will develop spiritually and become competent in a system of energy work. I don't support this dangerous dead-end street in any way. No one grows just by learning a technique or through an initiation. Only when a person uses these types of means in order to let qualities like love, consciousness, and personal responsibility grow within himself and these qualities are integrated into his everyday life through repeated new attempts, seriously and realistically confronting his fears and other blocks, does a person mature and become competent in relation to the use of such tools and imparting the corresponding knowledge to others. He has walked the path.

---

*This insight led to the development of Rainbow Reiki.

It is important to me to clarify that I principally have nothing against further initiations, symbols, rituals, mantras, and techniques of energy work, neither with regard to Reiki nor any other system as long as this is not supported by a superficial and "no-deposit-no-return" way of life that ultimately makes people sick. At the beginning of the Age of Aquarius, humanity is challenged to change our way of thinking. With consumption at any price and a technical-mechanical understanding of the world that considers goals more important than the paths with which they are achieved, we have ridden into ecological and social problems of gigantic dimensions. I think it is absolutely superfluous to also support such a mental attitude in the esoteric and spiritual area.

It is a paradox to collect initiations, degrees, and symbols in quick procession without taking the time to let the soul and the body grow into the tools—and at the same time claim that a person is holistically oriented and concerned with spiritual development. Growth needs time, personal commitment, the confrontation with competent teachers, a willingness to learn, and a great deal of courage to explore new shores and make real changes in the way of life. Initiations, mantras, symbols, and techniques of energy work are like good walking shoes, a backpack, and a cane—we make better progress with them, but we still have to walk.

Karuna Reiki

Primarily in America and England, a form of energy work is being taught under this name that is based on the initiation in four degrees dependent on each other (two Practitioner and two Master Degrees) with eight further symbols and teaching methods of their application within the scope of the energy work. The symbols have been channeled by various people, but belong to one system.

It was originally said that the Indian saint Sai Baba was the source of the messages and wanted to make Reiki more suitable for the New Age with them. Diverse inquiries at the Sai Baba organization could not verify these pronouncements, so that the founders of this method now assume that not Sai Baba but various subtle spirit guides and God himself are to be made responsible for the whole matter. This is why the Sanskrit work "Karuna"—the gist of which means: actions with which the suffering of other people is to be diminished—was introduced as the term to be used instead of "Sai Baba Reiki." In the initial period of this method's use, there were opinions that it was the original Usui system with the "genuine" symbols. These viewpoints also proved to be false. According to my research, the fact is that Karuna Reiki is a method of energy work based on initiation which functions with very good results, but actually has nothing in common with the Usui System of Natural Healing except the similar name: The initiation rituals, the energies employed, and the tradition differ greatly. It is good and useful when new forms of energy work are developed, but I think it is too bad that they usually do not have a name which clearly differentiates them from Reiki. Homeopathy and acupuncture are both wonderful healing methods. Because of the different names, every outsider also knows what is meant.

Foot Initiations

Through years of work, the Reiki Master, physical therapist, and practicing naturopath Gerda Drescher has developed a method of special energetic attunements (foot openings*) in connection with the long-term therapeutic measures of concretely improving her client's grounding. She has successfully employed this method since then and passes it on to her advanced students, who she also trains extensively in the related physical and psychotherapeutic accompaniment. She does not represent the standpoint that:

- the foot initiations are a component of the traditional Usui system.
- everyone who is initiated into Reiki automatically needs the foot initiations because the energy field of the body would become disharmonious or Reiki would not function properly.
- foot initiations are a "must" in the Age of Aquarius.
- grounding can only be achieved through foot initiations.
- foot initiations are appropriate for everyone.

---

*Foot openings are usually called foot initiations in informal language.

Quote: "Their (referring to foot initiations) effects have far-reaching consequences. In addition to an intensified connection to Mother Earth, this integration of the lower pole also leads to the confrontation with the physical nature, the unconscious mind, what is unredeemed within a person, and one's own shadow. They (the foot openings) are therefore in no way appropriate for filling a gap in the market and the pocketbook or polishing one's own ego, but require a process-oriented approach as well as accompanying responsible therapeutic know-how! I can make no statements about the effects of any other foot openings that someone claims to have received directed from a chosen Master or through meditation from Usui, the archangels, the Holy Spirit, and even God personally.

Although my foot openings have been developed in an intuitive, yet completely unspectacular empirical manner, and this is what makes them particularly valuable.

...Rei-Ki Balancing® is an invitation to connect more intensively with Earth Mother (Gaea) through one's own physical body and therefore requires taking the uncomfortable path from spirituality to wholeness as a process of individuation under the feet. ...Since I am convinced of the correctness and value of my work, I have worked out clear training structures and guidelines, the adherence to which can be controlled through the possibility of license revocation. The basic training lasts at least two to three years (depending on previous knowledge) and contains intensive and deep body work, among other things."

In accordance with the information I have, foot initiations according to Gerda Drescher (in connection with the therapeutic accompaniment she developed) are a completely respectable and effective method of healing grounding problems.

Is it Important to Have Both Hands Initiated into the Second Degree?

There are opinions that the three symbols and the mantras of the Second Degree should be given into both hands at the initiation into the Second Reiki Degree so that the symbols can be drawn with both hands and the Yin/Yang relationship remains balanced within a person. Is there something to this?

First, the good news: an initiation of both hands doesn't hurt anyone. However, it is not necessary. In the initiation into the Second Degree, the more mechanically skilled hand is initiated with the symbols and mantras because the signs can then be more easily practiced with pen and paper. The mechanically more skilled hand has the considerably better developed kinesthetic sense. The body movements are registered to the brain through it. So far so good.

Once the symbols and mantras are initially "inside" and a student of the Second Reiki Degree can draw them without errors by heart, it is usually superfluous to perform the signs by hand. The symbols and the mantras of the Second Degree are later primarily used in spirit by advanced Reiki students, except when it is a matter of refreshing the knowledge and exercising it. The Second Degree is a mental technique of energy work.

Since only the corresponding "tool kit" of symbols and mantras is made available for the Reiki students through the initiation, there will also be no displacement in the Yin/Yang relationship within the body during a correct traditional initiation. In my training practice with hundreds of Second Degree students, I have not observed any unnatural "masculinization," "intellectualization," or any other clear signs of a Yang imbalance—most of them are right-handed and receive the symbols in this hand as a result— through the Second Degree initiations. Since many of my students frequently come to my seminars as guests, even years later, and I receive news by letter and on the telephone about their developmental process, my experiences have a long-term background.

But as I said, it does not hurt anyone.

Chakra Initiations and Eye Initiations

Every part of an individual's body can fundamentally be initiated. Yet, in my opinion, this is not necessary. A type of energy tidal wave is sent through the organism in each initiation. With the corresponding personal preconditions, like the willingness to grow and heal, the energetic lever of a Reiki initiation—no matter what degree—can contribute some elements to a person's development. But you must still walk the path. Even if you have all seven main chakras initiated ten times a day into the Master Degree, you still have to go out into life. You cannot get around gathering experiences and struggling with the problems of everyday life. You must try time and again to learn from your errors and make the best of your weaknesses.

Last but Not Least . . .

When someone develops an initiation or energy-work method that makes it easier to work on real problems that could hardly be dealt with beforehand, I think this is very good. I find it even better if this person approaches the public without any masquerades and does not try to lure potential clients through promises that cannot be kept. Energy work of any type can help you walk the path if you have firmly decided to walk it and do your best. But energy work is not a computer-controlled "wheelchair to happiness." We are born on the earth to learn and to grow. This is only possible through acting with personal responsibility and constantly gathering and evaluating experiences.

Is There a Traditional Fourth Degree?

I myself teach and represent the Reiki path of three degrees. Still, I am also convinced that the Third Degree is not the final point of development in terms of initiations on the Reiki path. If a Master initiates another person to become a Master, because of this process he deals with a new energy quality, since he is a channel for the universal life energy. In my opinion, this process is comparable with an initiation that he himself receives.

The initiation of Masters used to be the special right of the Grand Master, since he was the only one to initiate others into the Third Degree. Since Phyllis L. Furumoto made this possibility available for all Reiki Masters who had already had some experience with the Third Reiki Degree some years ago, a "Fourth Degree" is basically open to all Masters who want to become involved in it and have worked with the Third Degree for some time. The essential learning processes of this degree probably relate to the stability in regard to one's own path since it is a part of the Master training for the student to clash with his teacher.

If the teacher is not stable and lets himself be made to feel insecure by the questions and reactions of his student, he cannot train others for the Third Degree in the long run since he would otherwise sway like a leaf in the wind. If he doesn't let himself be made to feel insecure, he cannot learn what he must learn. This "Fourth Degree" is then a constant balancing act. On the other hand, it is also a wonderful change for self-realization and helping others as well.

A good comparison depicting the character qualities required for the Third Degree training appears to be a bamboo plant. It is very strong, but can also bend when the pressure becomes too great. It can spring back when the pressure lets up. Its hull and roots are firm, but it is empty on the inside. In all structures it can still receive good things into itself and pass them on, if necessary. It is well-grounded and still light. Its growth is strong and straight, although it can sensitively sway in the wind.

In addition to the character qualities described, a Master who wants to train others must naturally have much experience with Reiki applications and himself have given a great many seminars on the First and Second Degrees. A good general knowledge of esoterics and the corresponding personal experiences are a part of this as well, as is at least fundamental knowledge about the structure and function of the human body.

Another very important point is money (once again!). A Reiki Master who cannot manage when it comes to the material realm, which means is not grounded in certain relationships, is not capable of imparting these experiences to others. If, for example, he is unable to fill his courses, he can hardly teach others to deal with this aspect of the Reiki Master work. If he still tries to train others in the Third Degree, clashes can quickly occur regarding participants when his student has also become a Master.

And this is perhaps even more important: If a training Master has financial problems, he can quickly be tempted to initiate a student even if he is not ready for it. This can bring great difficulties with it for the student's later work as a Master. In addition, it is a poor example that can have further disharmonious effects on other people in relation to their dealings with Reiki. The thought could very well arise that money is only important for the training Master, which is not true. This attitude could result in the conclusion of attempting to get the Third Degree initiation as cheaply as possible and miss the sense of this test. The path to becoming a Reiki Master would then not just be cheap in the material sense.

Now you probably think that Reiki Masters would be superior to such banal problems—but why should they be? Even someone who has been initiated into the Third Degree remains a human being!

Because the training to be a Master already requires a great deal of stability and a lot of personal experiences with Reiki, each Master should permit himself about three years of time after his own initiation into the Third Degree before he initiates others. In this way, he can learn to deal with the Master energy, the seminars, and questions by the students without immediately having to cope with the adventure of "Master initiation." Time is a very important factor in personal development—in the Third Degree as well. Although Reiki is immediately there when a person becomes initiated, the physical and mental structure needs a certain amount of time to open up to the new vibration and then re-orient itself.

Discount Master Trainings

There are currently many opportunties to get a title as cheaply and quickly as possible. However, a person who wants to *be* a Master needs time, commitment, and solid, comprehensive training—and something like this has its price. If you are considering aspiring for the Third Degree, give some serious thought to what is *really* important to you: appearance or reality!

So—this is the entire Reiki path. At least, it is the part of it that I have seen and become familiar with. I have given a detailed description of some aspects because I believe that this is important. Others, like this chapter for example, are shorter. First, because there are not so many people who actually gather practical experiences with the Third and "Fourth" Degrees. Secondly, because precisely this portion of the Reiki path has so many individual variations that an enormous amount could be written about it—or nothing at all. I hope that you have found a great many ideas for yourself and visualize a somewhat clearer view of the possible path of self-discovery with Reiki in front of your inner eye.

In order to once again give you a brief summary of the entire path of the Third and/or Fourth Degree and make the red thread a bit more visible, I have written the following chapter. You just need to keep on reading.

Chapter Seven

Once Again:
Reiki as a Path of Self-Discovery

You now have a bit more clarity about Reiki, the path of healing love. In the last chapters, a great many details about the degrees, their developmental possibilities, and the abilities that they contain have been portrayed. Perhaps your head is buzzing now from all the information and the questions which have (hopefully) been triggered in your mind.

In order to let the red thread that goes through the various degrees now become more visible, here is a summary of the essential points included in the Reiki path.

The Degrees

You become a Reiki channel through the initiations into the First Degree, which must be done by a traditionally trained Reiki Master. There are three different degrees in the Usui System of Reiki: the First Degree in which the fundamental abilities for the channeling of the universal life energy, as well as certain automatic protective mechanisms against the undesired transmission of personal energy through the Reiki channel and the Reiki recipient, are imparted. Once the abilities have been conferred, they remain a part of the initiated individual's personality forever. There are no possibilities of losing these abilities or artificially removing them. The Second Degree expands and supplements the knowledge gained in the First Degree with the "tools" of energy intensification, distance transmission, distance communication, and mental healing. An initiation and certain symbols and mantras are necessary for the application of these methods, as well as knowledge of their proper use. The Third Degree is the Master Degree. The initiation and a special Master symbol and mantra necessary for this purpose, as well as certain rituals, make it possible to be open to all living beings as a Reiki channel.

If a Reiki Master initiates another person into the Third Degree, a further process similar to initiation also occurs within himself. Once initiations have been given, they can never again be rescinded. Reiki in no way limits the individual's freedom to make decisions.

Reiki as a Path of Self-Discovery

Similar to Zen, Yoga, Tai Chi Ch'uan, and other methods for personal development, Reiki can be a path of spiritual self-discovery. The decision in favor of this must be made by each person on his own. If Reiki is "just" used as a holistic healing technique without the mental confrontation with one's own personal growth, the healing processes are then essentially limited to the physical level. Only the individual will for growth and direction of attention to the personal problem structures trigger mental and spiritual processes of development in correlation with regular contact with the universal life energy. These processes of development generally occur in accordance with a certain pattern (see chakra model, pg. 177) and in a specific rhythm.

How Reiki Stimulates Personal Growth

Reiki is a non-polar energy. The essence of this force is love. The processes which Reiki triggers always move in the direction of unity and harmony, which doesn't mean that unity and harmony will become manifest immediately after a Reiki session. It is up to every individual to accept unity and harmony or also resist it, which can cause feelings of suffering until the energy that has become conscious is once again suppressed or separated. If the power of love is accepted, the regular contact to the universal life energy creates relaxation, triggers detoxification processes on all levels, and then fills the person with clear, heavenly energy. Furthermore, the direction of attention to overcoming personal problem structures in connection with Reiki has the effect of orienting one's life within the scope of cosmic order (spiritual growth). Every degree offers new possibilities for this purpose, establishes new focal points, and permits the person to tackle his development from a different perspective each time, without making it impossible to do the work on the focal points of the previous degree at the same time. Each degree builds on the abilities of the previous one, but does not make them superfluous as a result.

Truth—Love—Perception

The development of the personality goes through three steps in each degree, as well as in each partial development of a characteristic in itself: truth, love, and perception. Through the process of relaxation, energies that have been previously suppressed can become conscious—a person learns more about himself. He sees a bit more of how he really is (truth). He doesn't have to like this truth. He can even hate this part of himself. However, in order to continue to grow he must learn to love this part, understand its meaning, and accept it. Through this process of loving and understanding acceptance, a weakness is transformed into a strength. Detoxification has taken place. The person has let more light into himself (love). The personality of the individual has become more complete. As a result, he can better fulfill his tasks in this life since he now has a greater range of possibilities available to him. He sees his relationship to the rest of the universe a bit more clearly and can bring his talents into the life processes of the totality. This process creates a far-reaching understanding of his self (perception), and therefore a transformation on a higher vibrational level.

The Personal Effort

In order to grow with the Reiki power, it is necessary to establish contact with it on a regular basis. This is possible through treatments and initiations into a Reiki degree. This contact makes the necessary amount and quality of energy available for the growth processes. How, where, and to what extent these actual developments are initiated is determined by the recipient since Reiki cannot trigger effects in a living being in contradiction to its deep-felt wishes. Instead of the conscious will, an orientation of attention towards a certain problem area is required.

The more a person is concerned with his shortcomings and at the same time has the wish to grow out of them, the more the regular contact with the universal life energy will set him into motion.

The Pleasure Principle and Harmonious Development

If the contact to Reiki is always sought when there is a desire for it, and it is not established when an emotional aversion to it exists, the development will take place harmoniously. If the Reiki sessions become an obligation, reactions of defiance and denial will occur, seriously obstructing the further development at some point. These reactions are caused by the Inner Child: Through the loving confrontation with its fears, it is possible to achieve a resolution of the attitude of denial, which is self-protection against the encounter with undesired emotional energies. Instead of discipline, loving consciousness work is then necessary to overcome the obstacles on the path. If parts of the personality and emotional energies are liberated through the Reiki work, it is quite possible that this process is felt to be a strain. In order to again feel a desire for further processes of development, it is necessary to have time, the confrontation with the purpose of the portions that have become conscious, and, if this is not enough, the gathering of experiences with the newly discovered aspects of the character in an environment that is protected and suitable for this purpose (self-discovery groups or something similar).

Reiki and the Processes of Becoming Conscious

All the "new" feelings, states of consciousness, and physical symptoms that have surfaced during the Reiki work also belonged to the person being treated before the session. However, they were not necessarily apparent because of suppression, projection, or separation. The contact with Reiki cannot create any truly new energies and structures, but just let those that existed latently now become conscious. It is then the individual's free decision as to how he will deal with the new portions of his personality, and whether he wants to learn to integrate them or seek new paths of suppression. Methods of psychotherapy or work in a self-discovery group can, in addition to other approaches, be very helpful in the integration work.

Complementary Methods of Opening Up to Reiki

In order to make it easier for the Inner Child to open up to Reiki, it is helpful to give it the opportunity of playing and satisfying its curiosity whenever this is possible. Instead of dogged self-discovery discipline, pleasure-oriented and alternating occupation with the body and the spirit should be placed in the foreground. Instead of constantly doing the same physical exercises, new ones can be tried out—alone or in a group, which is even better. Celebrating, dancing, and laughing are some of the most effective exercises to make the meaning of growth towards liveliness comprehensible to the Inner Child and awaken its desire. If the Inner Child finds no pleasure in growth, there will also be no true development in the overall personality of a human being!

All spiritual paths can enrich the Reiki path and accelerate the development on it. Reiki includes everything; it also intensifies and complements other methods of self-discovery. It knows no bounds and fundamentally obstructs no other energies since its quality is non-polar.

The Meaning of the Degrees

In contrast to other methods of personality development, on the Reiki path the contact to the energy and the use of the methods of dealing with it are always at the beginning of each section of the path. As an example of this, a Tai Chi student must practice intensively for many years in order to truly be able to work with the Ki and experience its effects. During this time, he learns much about himself and the work, going through many processes of development as a result.

A Reiki student visits a weekend seminar and can then already work successfully with Reiki. His growth process is now just starting. The situation is similar with the Second Degree and essentially with the Third Degree as well. We receive an ability that makes further learning possible for us. The Reiki path is not hierarchic, like the Tai Chi path, for example, but tends to be more holographic. From every standpoint, each type of personal development is principally possible, whereby the higher degrees with their expanded possibilities of dealing with Reiki make many growth processes easier. In strict terms, a Reiki degree says nothing about the personal maturity of the initiated since it is up to each individual to decide whether, how, and at what speed he grows. The Reiki degree only expresses something about the possibilities for channeling the Reiki power. The system of degrees thereby offers all people with their various personality structures a place from which they can have experiences with liveliness, love, and development, without being constricted in their personal freedom of decision.

The Type and Speed of Personal Growth

The quickest mental and emotional developments usually take place at the beginning of the work with a Reiki degree. Later, more personal effort that must take place in the form of directing the attention is required in order to set further processes into motion. This phenomenon can be explained with the pyramid model of personal structures. There are some problem structures at the very top that have been at the focal point of attention for a long time, even if this attention has not always been consciously directed. Often, the only thing missing to resolve them is vital energy. Through initiation into a Reiki degree or intensive Reiki sessions, this energy is made available.

The development process, for which the body, mind, and soul of the affected person have been prepared for a long time but could not be set into motion because of a lack of energy, then takes place very quickly. The underlying layers of our personality must once again be prepared for a resolution that can be cleared away by a renewed burst of energy. This preparation can be made through work on consciousness, direction of attention, or also through the pressure of suffering.

In the first two cases, a more intensive dissolution of the problem fields in general takes place quite harmoniously, but very challenging situations can occur on the basis of the latter situation. Here lies the deeper meaning of a conscious way of life. It facilitates holistic healing reactions. If the increasingly deeper-reaching healing process of the overall personality takes place gradually, the problem structures become increasingly subtle. A constant increase in sensitivity is necessary in order to direct the attention to the disharmonies. At the same time, the increased sensitivity is also disturbed by the personal process of growth.

The Steps of Growth

The changing topics of the problem areas can be explained through the chakra model. At first, those difficulties that relate to survival are clarified in one area (first chakra), then those of joy in life (second chakra), power (third chakra), love (fourth chakra), self-presentation (fifth chakra), and finally, those related to the perception of the self-realization for one's own path within the scope of the cosmic plan (sixth chakra). This means: Before you start building a cathedral, you first have to learn to lay bricks.

In this process, two topics that lie on an energetic plane form a structure with differing polarities (Yin and Yang). One of these topics tends to be accepted, and the other tends to be rejected. The state of tension developing between these poles triggers the growth pressure, which at some point leads to a merging of opposites on a higher plane. According to the order of development, here are the pairs belonging to each other: survival/joy in life: joy in life/survival; power/love; love/power; self-expression/perception of one's own path in the cosmic context; perception of one's own path in the cosmic context/self-expression. The term that is respectively listed as the first of a pair is the one that we tend to accept, while the one in the second position is the one we tend to reject.

Once we have gone through such a theme cycle in relation to a problem structure, it starts over again in the next problem structure, but on a higher level. The development takes place in the form of a double spiral (pairs of opposites), so that a theme that already had its turn "further down" must be dealt with at some later point again on a higher level.

This process of growth can be continued into eternity and on all levels of existence. This is life. Through its unity-promoting quality, Reiki stimulates the union of a pair of opposites on a respectively higher level of development. Directing the energy to a pair of opposites occurs by way of focusing attention.

Here is one example of this model of growth: A person who has to work twelve hours a day in order to just barely make a living (first chakra) becomes quite cross when his son doesn't even work the whole day, parties with friends, goes to the movies, spends time with his girlfriend, etc. (second chakra). The young man in turn is annoyed by the perpetual drudgery of his father, his monotonous and tedious way of describing his strenuous everyday life, and doesn't want to deal with this aspect of life at all.

This little example contains two successive tension patterns at the beginning of a cycle of growth. If you like, consider where such tensions occur in your life, what causes them to be resolved, and what new patterns then arise.

Situations of Illumination

So-called illumination always takes place when we succeed in putting ourselves into a state of being truly without any intentions. For a moment, we then find ourselves outside of this growth spiral with its development-promoting tensions. We do not desire to have the opposites resolved at this moment because we have taken a mental standpoint in which developments are not possible. Here is true unity, since all the energies are together here, in contrast to the apparent unity when a person has achieved a developmental step by unifying a pair of opposites. Then there is unity only in relation to these two energies.

Through the constant growth process in which we find ourselves, the next polarity is already programmed in advance and we still find ourselves on the development spiral. Illumination can then be achieved from any situation in life and at every level of development. It does not represent the final stage of a development but the suspension of all growth processes for a short period of time. A state of illumination promotes later developmental processes that are engaged in after the mental return to the spiral since the conscious experiencing of the unity creates a different, more relaxed approach to tension situations produced by the opposites.

The union of opposites is promoted by the experience of observing the spiral from the outside that has now been experienced. Then everything tends to be more an exciting game than dead earnest once you have looked backstage at the theater and know that all the stage sets are only made of paper maché and all the weapons of soft rubber.

Reiki and Illumination

Through the quality of unity, the Reiki power is basically an "energy of illumination." For people who have consciously or unconsciously opened up to it, the intensive contact with Reiki during an initiation or a longer treatment can also contain an experience of illumination. Contact with Reiki that is frequent, conscious, and without any expectations therefore generally supports development and a relaxed, more free approach to all situations in life. Tensions are then released more quickly and easily, and developmental steps taken more playfully.

Postscript

This chapter is not necessarily all that easy to comprehend. In case there was one thing or another that you didn't understand right away, simply let the information and thought-provoking impulses take effect for a while and then read the chapter again. Look for examples in your own life that will help you gain access to this topic. I've tried my best to treat it in a brief and understandable manner, but its nature can bring some difficulties in communication along with it. Although this chapter is quite theoretical, it can have enormous effects on your way of life and how you deal with Reiki if you examine it closely. Try it!

Chapter Eight

Reiki Resonance Therapy

A great hurdle, not just on the Reiki path, is a person's lack of ability to resonate. This problem manifests itself in such a form that energetic therapies of all types, such as Bach Flowers, homeopathy, Reiki, or shiatsu, show hardly any or no effect at all, even though they are competently applied. Subtle energy fields cannot be perceived, or only vaguely, although the respective person has invested a great deal of effort in the corresponding exercises. There may also be a strong insensitiveness in relation to one's own feelings or those of other people, in addition to a distinct inflexibility. Illness tends to take a chronic course, and it is difficult to learn from errors.

In homeopathy, where this syndrome has also been familiar for a long time, it is recommended that a so-called reaction remedy, such as Sulphur, Silicea, or Magnesium Fluoratum, be given in such cases along with a purification diet.* There are various possibilities available in Reiki therapy, which naturally should be supported by an appropriate diet as well. I would like to briefly introduce some of them here:

1. Reiki whole-body treatments

It is best to do a longer series of consecutive whole-body treatments daily or at least every second day in order to raise the overall vibrational level and help the body expel or transform energies and substances that obstruct its ability to resonate. The effect can be seen in the improvement of the symptoms listed above, in addition to the healing reactions familiar from all holistic therapies. This classic method functions quite well, but it can sometimes be very time-consuming in obstinate cases. The reactions

---

*Refer to the chapter on this topic in my book *Reiki for First Aid*, Lotus Light.

that occur in the process can turn out to be quite intensive andunpleasant, although they naturally contribute to the body, mind, and soul once again becoming more lively and happy.

2. Reiki whole-body treatments combined with special positions

This procedure is different from the one described in the previous point only in that the main detoxification organs—liver, spleen/ pancreas, kidneys, intestines, and the large lymph nodes—are additionally provided with an extra portion of Reiki. Instead of the usual three minutes per position in the whole-body treatment, at least 10 minutes should be planned. In this manner, the toxins and waste products create less congestion in the arterial roads of the body and elimination takes place in a considerably more harmonious manner in many cases. This method is based on the classical detoxification programs of natural healing therapies in which therapies for the detoxification apparatus are administered to stimulate elimination. The disadvantages here are the relatively large expenditure of time and the need for the Practitioner to have extensive knowledge of natural healing therapies so that a truly accurate diagnosis as to which detoxification organs function adequately and which ones need to be strengthened additional can be given in difficult cases. The techniques of the Second Degree can be a great help here. If, for example, the Inner Child and the Higher Self of the client additionally receive Reiki, these archetypical partial personalities can do their part in order to let the healing process occur more harmoniously and effectively. Through the Reiki mental healing with selected affirmations (see Chapter Four), the habitual patterns that obstruct healing or allow new problems to arise can be resolved in a specific and natural manner.

3. Reiki whole-body treatments combined with other holistic therapies

Here as well, the foundation is a series of whole-body treatments. In addition, the appropriate homeopathic remedies, flower essences, Aura Soma, phytotherapy, acupuncture, shiatsu, or a Mayr cure, and naturally psychotherapeutic measures can also be applied. In my experience, this procedure is particularly suited for naturopaths and doctors who treat with natural healing therapies since it obviously requires the relevant professional knowledge.

4. Reiki resonance therapy

I developed this method because it appeared important to me to work out an application that non-professionals can also use and is both effective and as gentle as possible. At the same time, it is suited for treating difficult cases in addition to professional medical care. It is also beneficial for people who simply want to do something for their personal and spiritual development but don't have any greater difficulties to deal with. For ideas, I turned to friends and teachers who work shamanically, studied the Filipino healings and ancient Polynesian Huna system of energy work and holistic healing. After becoming thoroughly familiar with the topic, I soon developed three important perceptions:

a. For reasons unknown to me, the joints are often used for depositing substances and subtle energies that the body can neither detoxify nor eliminate at the moment. The more the joints are blocked in one way or another, the more difficult it is for the organism to detoxify itself on all levels. The result is that it becomes less flexible.

b. The back in general and the part of the bladder meridian that goes through it is particularly favored as the "final disposal site" for the soul's garbage, the non-integrated experiences, the unhealed emotional injuries, and the like. In the course of time and naturally dependent on the amount and intensity of the suppressed experiences, considerable tensions of the back musculature can arise as a result of this. Late symptoms of this can then be damage to the posture, problems of the spinal column, and disorders like the shoulder-hand syndrome.

c. If, over a longer period of time, a person hates, cannot forgive, grieves, is envious, feels afraid, jealous, or greedy for something that he cannot have, he will poison himself mentally and emotionally. Later, this also manifests itself on the physical level itself and he loses his softness, liveliness, and ability to adjust, which means that he also suffers a drastic reduction of his flexibility.

The Reiki resonance therapy accordingly consists of three applications that complement each other. First, the joints of the body are supplied with Reiki. As in the whole-body treatment, about three minutes per position are enough for this purpose. The following suggested sequence has proved to be most effective after many experiments. At the same time, the sky won't fall down if you do it differently. In any case, in my extensive treatment practice I haven't experienced any greater problems caused by another sequence. But in difficult cases I suggest applying the methods explained here to be on the safe side. Perhaps in time you will develop even more effective applications in general or for special cases. I would be very pleased in this case, as I would also be to receive reports of experiences with this treatment.

Preparation: Smooth out the aura from the head to the feet a number of times.

1. Toes (including the base of the toes!)—2. ankles—3. knees—4. sacrum—5. hip joints—6. one hand on the sacrum, the other on the somewhat protruding vertebra at the base of the neck. If possible, these positions should be provided with Reiki for twice as long, which means about six minutes. —7. finger knuckles—8. finger joints (connective joints between fingers and hand)—9. wrist joints—10. elbows—11. base of the upper arms (connective joint between arm and shoulder)—12. shoulder blades—13. cervical vertebra (including the first cervical vertebra)—14. jaw joints—15. upper side of head.

Conclusion: Smooth out the aura from the head to the feet a number of times.

164

This part of the treatment should be given daily for about one week and even longer in serious cases. If you don't have any special problems, one treatment every 14 days is enough. More than this naturally doesn't hurt. Reiki will now slowly promote the functioning of the joints on the energetic level and initiates an intensified metabolism. This will improve the exchange of energy with the environment. Grounding and connection to spiritual powers are supported to the same extent. Furthermore, it creates the precondition for the gentle reduction of blocks in the back area.

The following application should be done directly after the previous one:

Use positions 1 to 6 as in the first part of the Reiki resonance therapy. Then, treat the area next to the spinal column beginning at the shoulders—handbreadth by handbreadth—down to and including the buttocks. Hold each position for at least three minutes.

It is strenuous to hold these positions for yourself with the First Degree, so please ask a Reiki friend to do it for you. If you have learned the Second Degree, you are naturally not subject to this restriction and can do it for yourself without any problem in this case.

Only do the first two treatments on consecutive days. Then, always have a pause of two to three days between the sessions. A total of about 10 to 12 of these treatments should be given. If there are no particular problems, then one to two times a month should be enough.

The following application can already be started after the first two sessions of the last partial treatment. Take about 20 minutes a day to do this for one week, and look for a place where you will be undisturbed during this time. After the first week, it is enough to carry out this Reiki ritual every 5 to 10 days. If you have no problems of a serious nature you would like to work on, once every four to six weeks is enough. When you do this, light a candle and an incense stick, preferably with sandalwood or frankincense:

- On a piece of paper, write down everyone you hate or cannot forgive for whatever reason. Put your hands on the third and the sixth chakra. Let Reiki be absorbed for a moment and say: "I ask the creative power ... (add your name here) to learn to forgive these people." Give yourself Reiki on your heart for a moment before starting the next step.

- On a piece of paper, write down everyone and everything you still mourn about. Put your hands on the third and sixth chakra. Let Reiki be absorbed for a moment and say: "I ask the creative power ... (add your name here) to heal my sadness, understand the meaning, and find fulfillment and joy in the present." Give yourself Reiki on your heart for a moment before starting the next step.
- On a piece of paper, write down everyone and everything you are envious about. Put your hands on the third and sixth chakra. Let Reiki be absorbed for a moment and say: "I ask the creative power ... (add your name here) to teach me to satisfy my true needs on my own and to heal my envy." Give yourself Reiki on your heart for a moment before starting the next step.
- On a piece of paper, write down everything that you afraid of. Put your hands on the third and sixth chakra. Let Reiki be absorbed for a moment and say: "I ask the creative power ... (add your name here) to teach me to find my inner strength and use it in the sense of life and love. I ask for the healing of my fears." Give yourself Reiki on your heart for a moment before starting the next step.
- On a piece of paper, write down everything that makes you jealous and everyone you are jealous of. Put your hands on the third and sixth chakra. Let Reiki be absorbed for a moment and say: "I ask the creative power ... (add your name here) to teach me to recognize and satisfy my true needs. I ask for the healing of my jealousy." Give yourself Reiki on your heart for a moment before starting the next step.
- On a piece of paper, write down everything you are greedy for. Put your hands on the third and sixth chakra. Let Reiki be absorbed for a moment and say: "I ask the creative power ... (add your name here) to teach me to recognize and learn to satisfy my true needs. I ask for the healing of my greed."*

---

* In case you should wonder similar formulations are used for the healing of envy, greed, and jealousy: these three character weaknesses all have the same background. There is a great inability to perceive the true needs and satisfy them on the basis of personal responsibility. Give yourself some minutes of Reiki on your heart before you end this Reiki ritual.

Slowly and consciously take the entire paper and burn it in a fire-proof container. Look at the flames and say: "My my errors and weaknesses are now healed. May I grow in the ability to understand and learn to love myself like I am."

This part of the Reiki resonance therapy is very intensive, which is why I have put it at the end of the overall treatment. The inner willingness to work through emotional problems is frequently lacking until at least the first part of the Reiki resonance therapy has been carried out.

Don't plan on doing anything that causes stress directly after this exercise.

It is not absolutely necessary to always use all three parts of the Reiki resonance therapy. Experiment with these treatment methods and convince yourself of their effectiveness. They can be employed in a great variety of ways and have already created a solution in some difficult cases. If you have the feeling during the treatment with the second part that it is appropriate to once again fit in some sessions with the first part, do it. The same naturally applies to the third section as well. Supplementing it with the Second Degree techniques, like Reiki contacts with the Inner Child and the Higher Self, karma-clearing, or also Rainbow Reiki, can effectively support the progress of the healing.

Although the Reiki resonance therapy is healing in a variety of respects, it cannot and should not replace the "usual" whole-body treatment. It is meant to be a way of opening and a revealing means of supporting the willingness to heal and ability to resonate.

The Reiki resonance therapy generally has a comparatively gentle effect. This is also one reason, among others, why I developed it. However, if greater emotional problems should arise, take advantage of the help of a psychotherapist. For serious physical problems, you should consult a medical doctor who works with methods of natural healing.

Chapter Nine

Professional Standards for Reiki Training Courses*

Because of the enormous amount of Reiki seminars offered, it is not always simple for an outsider to judge what contents this type of training should absolutely include, meaning which of the arrangements offer what is definitely necessary for an introduction to the Usui System of Natural Healing.

In this chapter, I would like to present what I feel to be the fundamental contents of training for the three traditional Reiki Degrees, as well as ethical guidelines for the work as a Reiki Master, both in the form of checklists. These standards are the result of my nine years of experience in the Reiki scene (as of 1996) and work with more than 3,500 participants in my seminars and workshops.

If you are thinking about participating in Reiki training, you can compare the various offers on the basis of the checklists.

If you are a Reiki Master yourself, with the help of the checklists you can examine the level of your knowledge and perhaps find a new personal relationship to your responsibility as a Reiki Master by reflecting on the ethical guidelines. If you already know and can do all of this or even more—then so much the better. Share this with your seminar participants and make it public! Talk to your colleagues about it. You will certainly contribute to raising the general level of quality.

It's too bad that advertising for most Reiki seminars is done with just an indication of the date and time, place, and price, as well as the name of the Reiki Master. When more information is given on the contents of the courses, it is easier for interested individuals to choose what is appropriate for them.

I generally differentiate between the basic training in the First, Second, and Third Degrees and advanced courses on each of these.

---

* The original version of this text was published in the magazine "Connection," edition 2/94. An expanded and revised version then appeared in the "Reiki Calendar 1996," publisher: Andrzej Bukowski, edition treve. I have once again revised and updated the current version.

In many seminars today, basic training is already combined with advanced training so that contents extending beyond the traditional Usui System are taught additionally. I also do this because I enjoy going on journeys of discovery together with the participants and living out my playful instincts.

Since almost every Reiki Master has developed his own applications on the basis of the Usui System, it is difficult to compare them. If one person includes meditation in the training for a degree and the other teacher uses healing stones or Bach Flowers, we cannot say which approach is better or worse. And this certainly is not what's significant. It's important to understand your own wishes and attend a Reiki seminar that satisfies these as completely as possible, as well as one that offers a proper introduction to the method itself. The checklists included below have been developed for this purpose. Talk with the respective Master about his individual program and let it be explained to you. In addition to such combined seminars, there are naturally also straight basic courses which contain little or no advanced material. This way of teaching and learning Reiki also has its appeal.

In my opinion, a development that has long been due in the Reiki area is one in which Reiki students learn from various Masters in order to be exposed to the enormous spectrum of this art. In other spiritual traditions—such as Zen, Tai Chi Ch'uan, or shiatsu—this has been common for many years. Go ahead and grant yourself a number of First Degrees, naturally with an adequate amount of time between them, with different Reiki teachers and carefully select what interests you from the many offerings. It is certainly worth investing a bit of effort in the planning of the path. Furthermore, the anticipated pleasure increases when you do this.

Reiki Checklist I

Here are the minimum requirements in relation
to the contents of a First Degree Reiki seminar:

The time-frame of the seminar: 2 days or about 12 hours of
instruction, not including the breaks. As an alternative to
this, four consecutive evenings, mornings, or afternoons are
possible:

Initiations: a total of four initiations, with a maximum of two per
day and at least three hours between them, should be given.
The greatest length of time from one initiation to the next
should not exceed more than 24 hours. If the initiations into
the First Degree take place with considerably more time between them, their effectiveness can no longer be ensured.

Religion or religious persuasion: These are not to be dictated.
Reiki is independent of definitive world views and not connected with any religion.

The history of Reiki: The history of the Reiki method (precise
name: Usui Shiki Ryoho, which is translated to mean the Usui
System of Natural Healing) should be told starting with Dr.
Mikao Usui, its founder in our age, and up to the present day
so that participants can become familiar with the tradition along
whose lines they are being trained. In addition, the Reiki history offers the opportunity of many important ideas for personal development and a meaningful approach to Reiki.

Reiki life principles: The five traditional life principles should be
taught, in addition to the history of their origin and their relation to the Reiki method, as well as an explanation of their
concrete use in relation to Reiki given. If the training Reiki
Master has developed further principles of his own, assumed
them from his own trainer, or reformulated the traditional principles, he will state this and explain the reason why he has
done so in order to give the students the possibility of their
own interpretations.

Reiki techniques: One form of the Reiki whole-body treatment
(head, front and back sides, legs, feet) in which all the vital
organs of the body, as well as the seven main chakras are provided with Reiki either directly or through reflexes. The par-

ticipants must have the positions demonstrated and related individual functions explained to them. There must be the opportunity for all those attending the seminar to practice. The exercises must be monitored and, if necessary, corrected by the training Master or a competent assistant whom he has selected.

Basic principles on the effect of Reiki: How does Reiki function in comparison to other methods of energetic healing? Which problems could arise from the increasing physical detoxification and the improved functioning of the organism in connection with the administration of medications prescribed by a doctor? What are the healing reactions in a holistic healing process? How can these be expressed in physical, mental, and emotional terms? How is Reiki used for chronic complaints and how is it used for acute complaints in order to have an optimum effect? How can the energy congestions that arise during the treatment be eliminated? What are the limitations of Reiki treatment for non-professionals? What is the task of energy exchange within the scope of holistic healing?

Laws pertaining to non-medical practitioners: The important contents of laws pertaining to non-medical practitioners (or the corresponding regulations in other countries) must be brought to the attention of the participants.

Responsibility: Elaboration on limitations in the treatment of serious physical or emotional disorders by non-professionals, explained on the basis of practical examples. Participants must be informed that trained medical professionals are always to be consulted in the cause of doubt and that non-professionals are not permitted to make any form of diagnosis or prescribe therapies. The legal and ethical grounds for this must be presented. It is irresponsible to promise healing. Other people should not be treated without their permission.

Seminar material: Written accompanying material on all important topics of the seminar is distributed without any further costs to the participants.

Reiki Checklist II

The time-frame of the seminar: At least one evening and one day or about 9 hours of instruction. As an alternative, the seminar can be held on three or four consecutive evenings, mornings, or afternoons.

Initiations: One initiation into the three Second Degree symbols and the related mantras.

Reiki techniques: Distance healing as self-treatment and for the treatment of other people; group distance healing; mental treatment with physical contact and within the scope of the distance treatment, with affirmation and without affirmation. Explanation of the difference between suggestive or hypnotic use of affirmations and the different function of affirmations within the scope of Reiki mental healing. Room purification and energy intensification of the Reiki flow. All techniques are theoretically explained and actually practised.

Symbols and mantras: The seminar participants must have all three symbols and their related mantras introduced to them, including an explanation of their fundamental translation from Japanese. (If this has given you a scare, don't worry: there are Japanese-English dictionaries that are suited for the translation of the Reiki mantras of all degrees.) The participants receive adequate opportunity to practice the symbols and mantras, learning them by heart. Even after the course, the trainer is willing to improve on any inadequate knowledge.

Responsibility: Distance treatments should only be given with the express permission of the client. Direct energy work on people without their express permission is an encroachment on their personal rights and has nothing to do with spirituality. The times for the treatments should be agreed upon for the purpose of achieving optimal results. For a mental healing, only use affirmations that have been agreed upon with the client.

Seminar material: Written accompanying material on all important topics of the seminar is distributed without any further costs to the participants.

Reiki Checklist III

The minimum requirements in relation
to the contents of a Third Degree Reiki seminar are:

Length: 12 months, then at least one year with the possibility of further supervision by the trainer if personal crises based on occupational changes are expected and gaps in knowledge become evident. This length of training time is necessary in any case in order to give the candidates for the Third Degree the opportunity for personal growth, the development of the Master personality, and the individual approach to the Reiki system. As soon as a person has decided on training in the Third Degree and has been accepted by a Master as a student, a subtle but lasting stimulation of personal maturity through the Reiki force begins. For this spiritual influence to have the best effect for the student, much time and commitment is necessary on the part of the student and on the part of the teacher. Based on my experience, training on one day, on one weekend, or for one week is in no way suited for imparting even an appreciable part of the technical or spiritual contents of a solid Third Degree training.

Initiations: One initiation into the symbol and the mantra of the Third Degree.

Reiki techniques: The four initiation rituals for the First Degree, the one for the Second Degree (three mantras and three symbols), and the one for the Third Degree are theoretically explained and actually practiced. The instruction on the initiation ritual for the Third Degree can also take place later, as soon as the training Master wants to train Masters personally.

Further training contents: Clarification of student's motivation for the Master training—group dynamics—extensive general knowledge of anatomy and physiology—assistance in at least 5 seminars on the First Degree and 5 seminars on the Second Degree—the teacher-student relationship from the psychological and spiritual viewpoints—information on taxation related to seminar income and on business expenses—economic and personal perspectives for self-employment—inner and outer structures of the initiation seminars on First and Second Degree Reiki—health and illness from the holistic perspective—taking inventory and initiating the therapeutic treatment of the Master student's personal problems, particularly his fears, claims to power, competitive structures, and learning inhibitions (sabotage programs) in the holistic sense—working through the currently available literature on the topic of Reiki—teachings about the aura and chakras, as well as principles for holistic personal consultation.

Training material: Written accompanying material on all important topics of the training seminars is distributed without any further costs.

Ethical Guidelines for Reiki Trainers (Masters/Teachers)

Live up to the responsibilities in the function of a trainer. Fulfill the obligation of constant continued learning in the professional field. Confidentially treat personal information from students. Only pass on what you understand yourself and master in the practical sense in your function as a trainer. Don't pull students into a personal dependence. Deal fairly and clearly with service and return service, energy exchange in general, and money in particular. Do not enter into any type of erotic or sexual relationships with students on principle. If this happens anyway, immediate make it clear to the student that the beginning of a partner relationship is the end of the teacher-student relationship; give yourself time to think about your own relationship wishes and point out the possibility of unclear transferences and counter-transferences in the psychotherapeutic sense.

No drugs before or during seminars or consultations! Avoid the creation of dependencies between teacher and student. Do not give the direct or indirect impression that happiness in life, success, wisdom, health, growth of the personality, and competence can be purchased in any of the Reiki Degrees per initiation. Personal opinions should be labelled as such. Make it clear that no "ultimate wisdom" can be imparted, but the respectively relevant level of perception in the professional area and the teachings that have been learned from personal experiences up to the present time. In the area of self-discovery, only convictions can be scrutinized and consciousness created. But every person must find and walk his path alone. Particularly during the first years of work, the trainer should engage in supervision sessions with a competent psychotherapist on a regular basis in order to perceive personal problems in the professional area in time and be able to provide therapy for them before his students must suffer as a result.

Special Guidelines for Reiki Masters
Who Want to Train Others
in the Master/Teacher Degree

Until personal competitive structures have been perceived and given fundamental therapy, seminars have been held over a longer period of time (at least one-and-a-half years—the more, the better—with about two well-attended seminars per month), and extensive competence has been achieved in the specific contents of the First, Second, and Third Degrees, a person should not attempt to train Reiki Masters. I also consider a longer period of psychotherapy (or a similar therapy) to attain clarity about one's own transference patterns and personal harmonies as absolutely necessary to prepare for the work as a Master trainer. If you want to train Reiki Masters/teachers, you should be clear about the responsibility associated with this work and fundamentally examine your motives. The wish to earn money should be at the bottom of this list. It is respectable to earn good money with good work, but when a person primarily works for the sake of money, the heart energy is lost from the work and then spirituality disappears as well. Work *with* money, but not *for* money. The same applies for the personal claims to power, which every trainer should be clear about. It is absolutely necessary to self-critically scrutinize one's own approach to power, fear, greed, and manipulation time and again; if necessary, work with a professional in the therapeutic field within the framework of supervisory sessions.

Short Introduction to Chakra Theory

Knowledge about the theory of chakras can help you better understand yourself, your life, and your development, making it possible for you to deal with yourself in a more harmonious manner. For this reason, I want to give a brief explanation of what chakras are and what functions they have.

What are Chakras?

A chakra (Sanskrit: wheel) is an energy center of the body that organizes certain life processes on the physical, mental, and emotional level. Clairvoyants see a chakra as a many-colored, rotating wheel.

In my vision of the theory of chakras (there are many others), I work with six main chakras and a seventh, the transformation chakra. In this context, I will not go into any further depth about the secondary chakras that also exist. Each chakra is connected with certain organs, sensory functions, parts of the body, and metabolic processes. At the same time, each of them represent one topic of personal growth.

Position and Tasks of the Main Chakras

You can see the physical position of the chakras in the adjacent illustration. Here are their names and fields of activity from bottom to top:

1. *Root chakra* (*topic:* survival, flight, preservation of the species, fight; *organs:* bones, nails, teeth, adrenal glands, legs, and everything solid within the body).

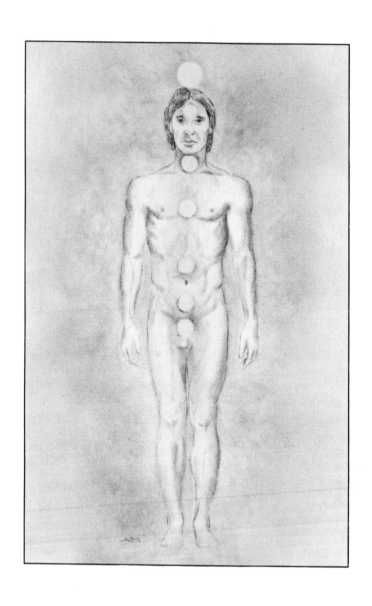

The seven main energy centers (chakras) of a human being

2. **Sexual chakra** (*topic:* joy in life, closeness, relationship, desire; *organs:* urogenital system, kidneys, skin, arms, and everything fluid within the body).
3. **Solar plexus chakra** (*topic:* power, domination, fear, karma, separation; *organs:* digestive system, liver, solar plexus, vegetative nervous system, joints, musculature's state of tension, energy metabolism, and detoxification processes through elimination/encapsulation).
4. **Heart chakra** (*topic:* love, unity; *organs:* heart, parts of the pancreas, thymus gland, detoxification processes through deposits in the fatty depot, and musculature's state of relaxation).
5. **Throat chakra** (*topic:* self-expression, individuality, communication; *organs:* neck, nape of neck, lungs, thyroid gland; equilibrium between physical and mental growth).
6. **Forehead chakra** (*topic:* perception of one's own path in the cosmic context; *organs:* ears, nose, eyes, and pituitary gland).
7. **Crown chakra** (*topic:* cosmic consciousness, transformation; *organ:* pineal gland).

According to my experience, the seventh chakra does not develop alone like the other chakras, but only when the blocks in the other chakras have been dissolved. Each time a person learns to love a little more, he comes a bit closer to God. This also sparks a developmental process in the seventh chakra. (Unfolding of the lotus with 1000 petals)

The first to sixth chakras are connected with each other in a great variety of ways. Here is a brief presentation of two of these connections:

1. The "hard" and the "soft" sequences:

In accordance with their characters, chakras one, three, and five are aggressive, dynamic—simply hard. Their comprehensive theme is "separation."

The characteristics of chakras two, four, and six are receptive, passive—simply soft. Their comprehensive theme is "unification."

A block in a hard chakra usually has an effect on the hard chakras that are further up as well. The same applies to the soft chakras.

2. The three levels of "earth—human being—heaven":

The chakras one and two can be classified on the level of "earth." Their tasks lie in the fundamental areas related to existence that make incarnation here on the earth possible in the first place.

The chakras three and four can be classified on the level of the "human being." The fundamental themes specific to human life occur here.

The chakras five and six can be classified on the level of "heaven." This is where the elementary spiritual growth processes occur that can bring the person in contact with the divine level, the level of unity.

Each level is built on the one below it. If the level of "earth" is not accepted and lived out, there can be no development on the level of "human being." If the level of "human being" is not accepted, there can be no development on the level of "heaven." If the level of "heaven" is not accepted and lived out, there can be no contact with God.

Chakras also cannot be "developed away." Aggression/survival, sexuality/joy in life, and power/dominance also have their place in spiritual growth, making it possible in the first place in a certain sense.

"Opening" the Chakras

"Opening" the chakras as a goal of personal evolution is often understood to mean that the chakras should really be open all the time. However, the state of constantly open chakras can have very disharmonious effects. The word "opening" is much more used to denote giving the chakras the opportunity of more extensive opening (receiving and transmitting more energy) through the dissolution of blocks and more extensive closing (letting less energy in and out).

The Energy Bodies and Their Relationship to the Chakra System

In addition to the chakras, the subtle portions of a human being also consist of energy bodies that touch all chakras and organize specific levels of the overall personality (see illustration). Clairvoyants see these energetic bodies as the aura around the material body. These bodies are:

a) *The ether body*, which is newly formed in each incarnation and contains the physical structure of a human being, his vital energy, his receptive and active abilities on the subtle levels (extrasensory perceptions and magic).

b) *The emotional body*, which contains our feelings and instincts. Emotional energies that are not lived out are reflected on it in the form of blocks.

c) *The mental body*, which contains all the logical processes of thinking, both the conscious and the unconscious. Reflexes and value judgments, moral concepts and dogmas have their "playground" here. The perceptions of the physical senses flow into here and are put to use.

d) *The spiritual body*, which is the level of a human being closest to God. Each individual being is connected with all other parts of the creation through this body.

Commented Bibliography

Reiki

"The Complete Reiki Handbook" by Walter Lübeck, Lotus Light Publications. A detailed introduction oriented toward the practice of Reiki healing. There is an extensive ABC of special positions, as well as advice concerning Reiki and medication, Reiki meditation, work with precious stones and aromatherapy.

"ReikiFor First Aid" by Walter Lübeck, Lotus Light Publications. Reiki Treatment as accompanying therapy for over 40 illnesses with a supplement on nutrition. Has grown out of years of Reiki practice, observing the many special usages that have developed for Reiki. Its crammed to the margins with new information on Reiki and nutrition, as well as Reiki combined with other natural healing methods.

"Empowerment Through Reiki" by Paula Horan, Lotus Light Publications. This is an important book about Reiki because it describes many of the ideas of holistic medicine in relation to Reiki.

"Abundance Through Reiki" by Paula Horan, Lotus Light Publications. A powerful, poetic evocation of true Self and Universal Life Force Energy. The book describes the 42 steps from Core Self to Core Abundance, creating richness within and without.

The Subtle Energy System

"The Chakra Handbook" by Baginski/Sharamon, Lotus Light Publications. This is an excellent work about the functions of the seven main chakras with many exercises, classification tables and thought-provoking ideas.

"The Body of Light" by Mann/Short, Charles E. Tuttle, Boston. This is a very interesting introduction to various ways in which the great spiritual traditions look at the inner energy system.

"Chakra Energy Massage" by Marianne Uhl. Lotus Light Publications. An unusual new presentation of Foot Reflexology. Offers us a deeper understanding of the relationship between spirit and body.

Simple, practical instructions for synthesizing Chakra balancing work with Foot Reflexology.

"The Metamorphic Technique, Principles and Practice" by Gaston St. Pierre and Debbie Boater, Element Books Ltd., and **"Metamorphosis—A Textbook on Prenatal Therapy"** by Robert St. John, self-published, are two books about a fantastic self-help method which you absolutely must read. Alone and in combination with Reiki, they will open up for new worlds you.

"The Secrets of the Soil" by Tompkins/Bird, Harper. Some years ago, Tompkins and Bird wrote the best-seller **"The Secret Life of Plants."** Their new book is perhaps even more important. Through correct behavior in terms of our nutrition, it shows us possibilities to help re-balance our planet's ecological system, as well as our own body and spirit.

"The Secret Way of Wonder" by Guy Finley, Llewellyn, Public., St. Paul. This book describes discovering the world with the eyes of a child and thereby making healing and growth possible.

"Life Energy" by Dr. John Diamond, self-published. This book discusses kinesiology in reference to acupuncture meridians, reflex zones for testing and treatment and shows an interesting correlation to biochemistry.

About the Author

Walter Lubeck is a renowned Reiki master, founder and director of the Reiki-Do Institute. He is a bestselling prolific author of classic works on Reiki, as well as books on other healing methods, such as work with Chakra balancing, pendulums, and auras. In the last years he has developed a method he refers to as Rainbow Reiki which includes an unlimited spectrum of applications like channeling, astral travel, making Reiki essences, therapy with precious stones, as well as personality development and wholistic enviromental protection. He has spent many years studying diverse martial arts, meditation, natural healing and energy work of all kinds. Walter Lubeck orients himself in his entire work toward three basic principles: support of personal individual responsibility, development of the ability to love, and conciousness expansion. His goal is to contribute to the betterment of the quality of daily life through spiritual knowledge and thereby to bring man, nature and God in harmony. He lives with his wife, the philospher and shaman Greta Bahya, and child in Weserbergland, Germany in a landscape filled with ancient power spots.

If you would like to contact **Walter Lübeck** and *The Reiki Do Institute*, please write to:

Windpferd Verlag
"Reiki – Way of The Heart"
Friesenrieder Straße 45
87648 Aitrang

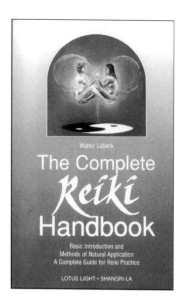

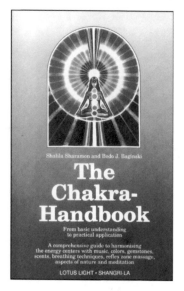

Walter Lübeck

The Complete Reiki Handbook

Basic Introduction and Methods of Natural Application – A Complete Guide for Reiki Practice

This handbook is a complete guide for Reiki practice and a wonderful tool for the necessary adjustment to the changes inherent in a new age. The author's style of natural simplicity, much appreciated by the readers of his many bestselling books, wonderfully complements this basic method for accessing universal life energy. He shares with us, as only a Reiki master can, the personal experience accumulated in his years of practice. Lovely illustrations of the different positions make the information as easily accessible visually as the author's direct and undogmatic style of writing. This work also offers a synthesis of Reiki and many other popular forms of healing.

192 pages, $ 14.95
ISBN 0-941524-87-6

Shalila Sharamon and Bodo J. Baginski

The Chakra Handbook

From Basic Understanding to Practical Application

Knowledge of the energy centers provides us with deep, comprehensive insight into the effects the subtle powers have on the human organism. This book vividly describes the functioning of the energy centers. For practical work with the chakras this book offers a wealth of possibilities: the use of sounds, colors, gemstones, and fragrances with their own specific effects, augmented by meditation, breathing techniques, foot reflexology massage of the chakra points, and the instilling of universal life energy. The description of nature experiences, yoga practices, and the relationship of each indiviual chakra to the zodiac additionally provides inspiring and valuable insight.

192 pages, $ 14.95
ISBN 0-941524-85-X

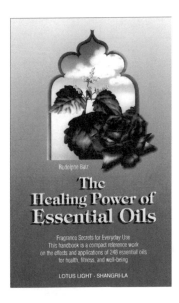

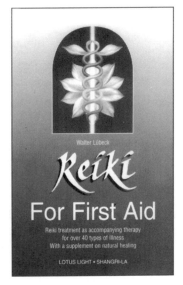

Rodolphe Balz

The Healing Power of Essential Oils

Fragrance Secrets for Everyday Use. This handbook is a compact reference work on the effects and applications of 248 essential oils for health, fitness, and well-being

Fifteen years of organic cultivation of spice plants and healing herbs in the French Provence have provided Rodolphe Balz with extensive knowledge about essential oils, how they work, and how to use them.
The heart of *The Healing Power of Essential Oils* is an essenial-oil index describing their properties, followed by a comprehensive therapeutic index for putting them to practical use. Further topics of this indispensible aromatherapy handbook are distillation processes, concentrations, chemotypes, quality and quality control, toxicity, self-medication, and the aromatogram.

208 pages, $ 14.95
ISBN 0-941524-89-2

Walter Lübeck

Reiki For First Aid

**Reiki Treatment as Accompanying Therapy for over 40 Types of Illness
With a Supplement on Natural Healing**

Reiki For First Aid offers much practical advice for applying the universal life force in everyday health care. The book includes Reiki treatments for over forty types of illness, supplemented with natural-healing applications and a detailed description of the relationship between Reiki and nutrition.
Reiki Master Walter Lübeck gives extensive instructions on topics ranging from Reiki whole-body treatments to special positions. These special Reiki treatment positions are an important contribution to the field of natural healing.

160 pages, $ 14.95
ISBN 0-914955-26-8

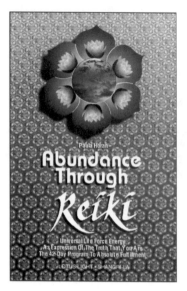

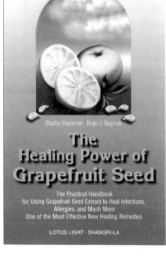

Paula Horan

Abundance Through Reiki

**Universal Life Force Energy
As Expression of the Truth That
You Are
The 42-Day Program to Absolute
Fulfillment**

Abundance Through Reiki is a powerful, poetic evocation of true self and universal life force energy. Its emphasis is a program of 42 steps from Core Self to Core Abundance, creating inner and outer richness. A detailed presentation in the form of two 21-day abundance plans takes you on an exploration of belief patterns that keep you from experiencing everything you need or desire.

Further topics are Reiki and abundance, abundance of health, love, friendship, knowledge, and experience. The book promotes your own natural ability to experience freedom, creativity, and authenticity.

160 pages, $14.94
ISBN 0-914955-25-X

188

Shalila Sharamon · Bodo J. Baginski

**The Healing Power of
Grapefruit Seed**

**The Practical Handbook for Using
Grapefruit Seed Extract to Heal
Infections, Allergies, and Much
More. One of the Most Effective
New Healing Remedies**

Latest scientific studies show that plant extract from grapefruit seeds has a large range of effects and applications for both internal and external use in preventative health care, therapy, cosmetics, and baby care. Based on international research, two bestselling authors have compiled sensational therapy successes and areas of application for this biological broad-spectrum therapeutic agent, antibiotic, antimycotic and antiparasitic, preservative, and hygienic agent of the future. In addition to scientific proof, this practice-oriented book includes proper dosages and procedures.

160 pages, $ 12.95
ISBN 0-914955-27-6

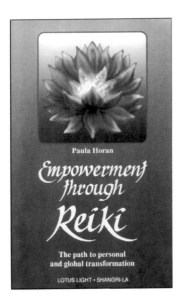

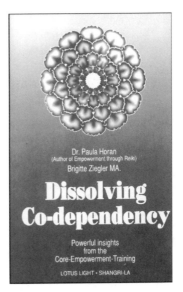

Dr. Paula Horan

Empowerment Through Reiki

The Path to Personal and Global Transformation

In a gentle and loving manner, Dr. Paula Horan, world-renowned Reiki Master and bestselling author, offers a clear explanation of Reiki energy and its healing effects. This text is a must for the experienced practitioner. The reader is leaded through the history of this remarkable healing work to the practical application of it using simple exercises. We are not only given a deep understanding of the Reiki principles, but also an approach to this energy in combination with other basic healing like chakra balancing, massage, and work with tones, colors, and crystals. This handbook truly offers us personal transformation, so necessary for the global transformation at the turn of the millennium.

160 pages, $ 14.95
ISBN 0-941524-84-1

Dr. Paula Horan · Brigitte Ziegler M. A.

Dissolving Co-dependency

Powerful insights from Core-Empowerment Training

Dr. Paula Horan, a noted American psychologist, and her partner Brigitte Ziegler, a well-known German seminar leader, are both Reiki Masters, well-versed in a wide variety of mind/body systems. They have put together a very powerful training program to assist people in the dissolution of a lifetime of inappropriate thought, emotional, and behavioral patterns. The ultimate necessity of "waking up" in its truest sense, gives very in-depth background to the real workings of the human mind. Each chapter is followed by a simple exercise to help the reader assimilate every area of understanding. This book is meant for people seeking greater knowledge about themselfs, with a sincere desire to get in touch with the core of their being.

102 pages, $ 9.95
ISBN 0-941524-86-8

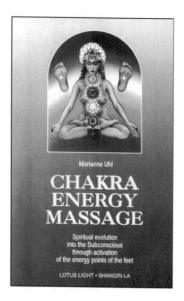

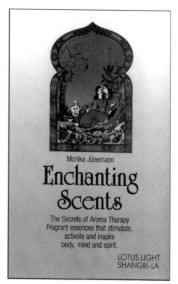

Marianne Uhl

Chakra Energy Massage

Spiritual Evolution in the Subconscious by Activating of the Energy Points of the Feet

This book guides you into the fascinating world of the energy body. Based on the knowledge of foot reflexology massage it introduces you to chakra energy massage, which can activate the individual energy centers of the human body. By means of the fine energy channels connecting them to the body's organs and energy centers, the feet reflect our physical and psychological condition. The author enables you to quickly acquire all of the knowledge needed for foot reflexology massage and chakra energy massage. In addition, she provides information on the vibrations of primal tones and various colors to effectively enhance your work with the chakras.

128 pages, $ 9.95
ISBN 0-941524-83-3

190

Monika Jünemann

Enchanting Scents

The Secrets of Aromatherapy Fragrant Essences that Stimulate, Activate and Inspire Body, Mind and Spirit

Today we are just as captivated by the magic of lovely scents and as irresistably moved by them as ever. The effects that essential oils have can vary greatly. This book particularly treats their subtle influences, but also presents and describes the plants from which they are obtained. It beckons you to enter the realm of sensual experience and journey into the world of fragrance through essences. It is an invitation to use personal scents to activate body and spirit. Here is a key that will open your senses to the limitless possibilities of benefitting from fragrances as stimulants, sources of energy, and means of healing.

128 pages, $ 9.95
ISBN 0-941524-36-1

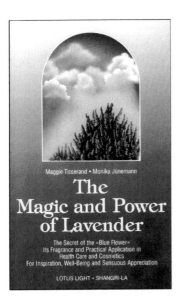

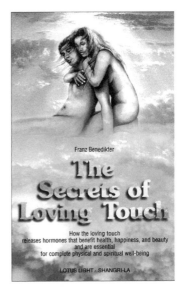

Magie Tisserand · Monika
Jünemann

The Magic and Power of Lavender

The Secret of the Blue Flower

The scent of lavender practically has permeated whole regions of Europe, contributing to their special character, and dominated perfumery for most of its history. To this very day, lavender has remained one of the most familiar, popular, and utilized of all fragrances.

This book introduces you to the delightful and enticing secrets of this plant and its essence, demonstrating its healing power, while also presenting the places and people involved in its cultivation. The authors have asked doctors, holistic health practitioners, chemists, and perfumers about their experiences and share them – together with their own with you.

136 pages, $ 9.95
ISBN 0-941524-88-4

Franz Benedikter

The Secrets of Loving Touch

How the Loving Touch Releases Hormones that Benefit Health, Happiness, and Beauty and Are Essential for Complete Physical and Spiritual Well-Being

Psychologist Franz Benedikter helps readers create the best possible hormonal basis for a healthy, happy, and liberated life. A release of relaxing, activating, and euphoretic hormones occurs when certain trigger zones of the body are gently touched. With this compact exercise program, we can have a positive effect on the body, mind, and soul through a form of self-massage and partner massage that is more like a loving touch. Since every healthy person has a longing to be touched, this book introduces a new age of tenderness.

144 pages, 12.95 $
ISBN 0-941524-90-6

ADDRESSES and SOURCES of SUPPLY

Fragrances, Gemstones, Herbs, Books and Cassettes

WHOLESALE

Contact with your business name,
resale number or practioner license.

LOTUS LIGHT ENTERPRISES, INC.
Box 1008 RWH
Silver Lake, WI 53170
Voice 414/889-8501 • Fax 414/889-8591

RETAIL

INTERNATURAL
33719 116th Street Box RWH
Twin Lakes, WI 53181